Promotion of Pharmaceuticals:
Issues, Trends, Options

Promotion of Pharmaceuticals: Issues, Trends, Options

Dev S. Pathak
Alan Escovitz
Suzan Kucukarslan
Editors

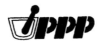

Pharmaceutical Products Press
An Imprint of The Haworth Press, Inc.
New York • London • Norwood (Australia)

Published by

Pharmaceutical Products Press, 10 Alice Street, Binghamton, NY 13904-1580 USA

Pharmaceutical Products Press is an imprint of The Haworth Press, Inc., 10 Alice Street, Binghamton, NY 13904-1580 USA.

Promotion of Pharmaceuticals: Issues, Trends, Options has also been published as *Journal of Pharmaceutical Marketing & Management*, Volume 7, Number 1 1992.

Library of Congress Cataloging-in-Publication Data

Promotion of pharmaceuticals : issues, trends, options / Dev S. Pathak, Alan Escovitz, Suzan Kucukarslan, editors.
    p. cm.
    Also published as Journal of pharmaceutical marketing & management, v. 7, no. 1, 1992.
    Includes bibliographical references.
    ISBN 1-56024-383-X (H : alk. paper).–ISBN 1-56024-384-8 (s : alk. paper)
    1. Drugs–Marketing. 2. Advertising–Drugs. 3. Pharmaceutical industry. I. Pathak, Dev S. II. Escovitz, Alan, 1947- . III. Kucukarslan, Suzan.
    [DNLM: 1. Advertising. 2. Drug Industry. 3. Drugs. QV 736P965]
HD9665.5.P76 1992
615'.1'0688–dc20
DNLM/DLC
for library of congress
          92-49617
          CIP

Promotion of Pharmaceuticals: Issues, Trends, Options

CONTENTS

ABOUT THE EDITORS

Dev S. Pathak, D.B.A., is Merrell Dow Professor and Chairman of the Division of Pharmaceutical Administration at Ohio State University. He has published over one hundred articles in peer-reviewed journals and is frequently invited to speak at national and international meetings on topics related to pharmacoeconomics, drug distribution and public policy, strategic planning and pharmaceutical organizations, and research methodology and pharmacy practice. He also holds a joint appointment as Professor of Marketing in the College of Business at Ohio State.

Alan Escovitz, Ph.D., is Director of Pharmacy Extension Services for the College of Pharmacy and Director of the Center for Continuing Health Sciences Education at Ohio State University. He is also Executive Director of the Council of Ohio Colleges of Pharmacy, the educational consortium of Ohio's four pharmacy colleges. Dr. Escovitz represents pharmacy on the Task Force on Industry/CME Provider Collaboration.

Suzan Kucukarslan, Ph.D., is Assistant Professor in the Division of Pharmaceutical Administration at the Ohio State University College of Pharmacy. Currently, her research interests include public policy and its impact on pharmaceutical industry, drug distribution and pharmacy practice, and consumer valuation of pharmacy services and drug products.

Pharmaceutical Promotion: Information or Persuasion?

Dev S. Pathak
Alan Escovitz
Suzan Kucukarslan

To promote is "to encourage the existence or progress of" an object, including a product, a service, an idea, or an organization. Thus, two major objectives of any promotional program are to inform and to persuade. Regardless, the desired endpoint of all pharmaceutical information is to facilitate rational decision making by all of the parties involved in the delivery and consumption of pharmaceutical care. Unfortunately, the second objective-to persuade a pharmaceutical care provider to select an advertised (or promoted) product-is frequently in conflict with the desired endpoint. Furthermore, the first objective-to inform-is now being questioned because of the commercial interests of a major source of pharmaceutical information, the pharmaceutical manufacturer.

The major informational effects of promotional programs are achieved by providing decision makers and/or consumers with information about the availability of pharmaceutical products, as well as other information about these products, so that they can make choices that reflect their preferences. Promotional programs that convey information are thus useful in assisting efficient market functioning and may result in stronger competition for both quality and price as well as stronger incentives for innovation. Modern economic theory also recognizes that the generation and dissemination of information is not free. Acquisition of information about pharmaceutical care by consumers or health care decision makers is costly. Hence, from an economic perspective, questions regarding

Dev S. Pathak, D.B.A., is Merrell Dow Professor, Alan Escovitz, Ph.D., is Director of Continuing Education and Adjunct Associate Professor, and Suzan Kucukarslan, Ph.D., is Assistant Professor, all at the Ohio State University College of Pharmacy, 500 West 12th Avenue, Columbus, OH 43210.

1

pharmaceutical information at the macro level relate to such issues as: Is pharmaceutical promotion excessive? Does the cost of pharmaceutical promotion put undue pressure on prescription drug prices? Do promotional expenditures by established pharmaceutical firms create barriers to entry for new firms and therefore reduce competition?

While the informational value of pharmaceutical promotion is less controversial among economists, it has been suggested that further regulations are needed to control the proliferation of misleading messages and to restrict the explicit and implicit persuasive powers of pharmaceutical promotion. Interest in these concerns has been further heightened since the publication of Food and Drug Administration (FDA) Commissioner Kessler's viewpoints on these issues in the 18 July 1991 issue of the *New England Journal of Medicine*. Traditional methods of drug promotion, such as print advertising, personal selling, and the distribution of detailing pieces at professional meetings, have been supplemented by new mechanisms of information dissemination, such as symposia and seminars, continuing health care education programs, and contemporary technologies such as audiovisual presentations on closed-circuit or cable television and interactive computer programs. The concern is not over the pharmaceutical industry's use of new information technologies, but whether these technologies are applied for the unbiased exchange of scientific information.

Dr. Kessler and the FDA are especially concerned with statements made by some researchers and medical experts at many of the industry-sponsored activities. Because of a possible relationship between industry sponsors and the expert speakers, statements made by these speakers can be construed as statements issued by, on behalf of, or under the control of the industry sponsor. To assist the pharmaceutical care provider in separating the promotional events (i.e., subject to FDA regulation) from nonpromotional scientific exchange (i.e., subject to First Amendment protection), Dr. Kessler has proposed at least four criteria that can be used to evaluate these industry-sponsored activities: independence, objectivity, balance, and scientific rigor. Using these criteria, the FDA issued a draft concept paper in October 1991 entitled, "Drug Company Supported Activities in Scientific or Educational Contexts."

While the FDA draft paper provides guidance on separating promotional programs from educational programs, Cooper suggests that the statutory authority of the FDA may not be as broad as construed by FDA officials. Readers are encouraged to compare the contrasting interpretations offered by Adams and Cooper of what is or is not promotional activity under the 1938 Food, Drug, and Cosmetic Act (FDCA).

In addition to the legal issues, the fundamental question in terms of pharmaceutical promotion is: What are the implications for public health and social welfare of strict interpretations of the laws regarding dissemination of information about pharmaceuticals? Keith proposes that answering this question requires balancing the cost of two types of errors associated with the regulation of information: allowing the dissemination of information that turns out to be false or misleading and restricting information that turns out to be true or highly valuable. As Keith points out: "If the information would lead a physician to know about a product that might be helpful for a few people in alleviating a mild symptom, the harm from not getting that information out is much less than the harm that might occur if the information is really true and would lead physicians to identify a remedy for a serious disease."

An interesting approach to weighing the benefits and costs of promotional programs and determining whether to enforce compliance through prosecution is adopted by the Federal Trade Commission (FTC) in evaluating misleading and/or deceptive advertising. The FTC approach is summarized in the *Cliffdale* case: ". . . the Commission will find an act or practice deceptive if first, there is a representation, omission, or practice that, second, is likely to mislead consumers acting reasonably under the circumstances, and third, the representation, omission or practice is material" [103 F.T.C. 165 (1984)]. This remark is clarified in this issue by Peeler's list of six criteria. Apparently, there is an implied theory underlying the FTC's approach consisting of constructs that can be used to determine how consumers are misled. A similar approach may be needed to describe and identify the determinants of misleading communications at industry-sponsored symposia for pharmaceutical products.

Such a theoretical framework could serve to identify those conditions, in addition to sponsorship by pharmaceutical manufacturers, under which a message may be construed as misleading. Alternatively, such a framework could assist in identifying those messages that are informational but fall within the category of unapproved labeling, such as educational activities related to unlabeled indications for anticancer agents. Understanding the major steps of information processing involved in the creation of misleading messages in receivers' minds may be one approach toward developing a theoretical framework. Without such a deductive framework, the FDA will continue to use its inductive approach to identify programs that are misleading, and controversies over what is promotional will continue. When finalized, the FDA draft guidelines may prove to be sufficient, since the FDA's interest is in identifying and preventing the transfer of misleading messages. However, this is not sufficient for industry sponsors or for marketing and/or social-science researchers interested in knowing why a specific message may be misleading for an intended audience.

Finally, while regulators are asked to weigh the societal welfare implications of the information sponsored by pharmaceutical manufacturers as described by articles in this publication, their opinions do not exonerate the pharmaceutical industry and health care experts from their responsibility to society. As pointed out by Chren, Waldholz, and Cearnal, there are promotional abuses in the pharmaceutical marketplace, and the line dividing pharmaceutical promotion and pharmaceutical education is obscure. However, as Ingram points out in his article, if the patient is put first and "the promotion is done responsibly through truth well told," maybe education and promotion can take place at the same time.

We sincerely hope that articles published in this collection, based on presentations made at the 36th Annual Ohio Pharmaceutical Seminar in Columbus raise our level of consciousness regarding many perplexing questions involved in evaluating pharmaceutical promotion in our society. Putting the patient first should be the common goal of regulatory control and those advocating the free flow of information in the pharmaceutical marketplace. What is needed is not an adversarial but a cooperative relationship between the FDA and the pharmaceutical industry to commit our limited health care resources to the provision of rational pharmaceutical care.

Trends In Advertising Pharmaceuticals: A Publisher's Perspective

William J. Reynolds

There are many different ways we gather information, such as touching or feeling an object, smelling perfume or cooking odors, or biting into something tasty. But the two principal ways in which we gather information through advertising are to hear it and see it. An advertiser, therefore, has primarily two ways to communicate information to you. He can tell it to you or let you read it. For maximum impact, an advertiser will use both approaches to convey his message.

I have been involved in advertising for 20 years, for the past 9 years as the publisher of a number of magazines that circulate to health care professionals. Most of my time has been spent with our pharmacy publication, *Drug Topics*. So my emphasis may be on pharmacy. However, I will try to mention other medical professionals as well.

My company is one of the largest publishers of professional health care publications, reference books, and other communications vehicles. The publishing industry is going through some significant changes now. Indeed, what's happening at my organization is what's happening in medical advertising today. For example, within our organization, we have divided into two distinct companies. One, Medical Economics Publishing, consists of all of the magazines and journals directed to health care professionals. The other company, Medical Economics Data, publishes directories and reference publications, such as the *Physicians' Desk Reference* (*PDR*), the *Red Book*, and the *Medical Device Register*, and is involved in other data-based ventures. Why the split? It is no secret that electronics offers new opportunities in communications, especially with reference information.

There are many different forms of advertising, including journals,

William J. Reynolds is Publisher of Drug Topics/Medical Economics, 680 Kinderkamack Road, Oradell, NJ 07649.

5

direct mail, billboards, newspapers, TV, radio, salespeople, newsletters, directories, reference books, electronics, and word of mouth. Research has shown that in the pharmaceutical industry, physicians and pharmacists responded this way when asked to list their most important sources of information (not necessarily ranked in order):

- Journals
- Continuing Medical Education Courses
- Conferences and Conventions
- Colleagues
- Directories and Reference Books
- Pharmaceutical Representatives
- Dealers and Wholesalers
- Government Bulletins/Literature
- Direct Mail from Pharmaceutical Companies
- Videotapes/Films
- Radio Networks
- Cable TV
- Study Clubs/Discussion Groups

Advertising to the physician has evolved from these simple print ads in the first issue of *Medical Economics* in 1923 (Figure 1) to the more creative and informative ads that we see every day, ads such as these that appeared in recent issues for the products Procardia®, Halcion®, and Lorelco® (Figures 2-4).

In 1990, there were more than 41,000 advertising pages in 83 physician publications that we audit, for an estimated total expenditure of $190 million. All of these ads were designed to create product or company awareness and, ultimately, to help the health care professional better serve and educate the patient.

In pharmacy, *Drug Topics* traces its roots back 134 years. Figures 5-7 provide sample ads from some 80 years ago. Compare this with the more creative advertising of today, such as the ads for Imodium® and Pepcid® shown in Figure 8. Spending for advertising in major pharmacy publications that we audit totaled $9 million. That advertising ran in ten magazines. Advertising to the pharmacist is becoming increasingly important, since he is evolving as the gatekeeper of our industry. The pharmacist is the health care professional with the most direct link to the consumer.

We have just looked at some journal ads. Now let's look at direct mail. Direct mail comes in many different formats, from the simple postcard to the traditional package to the more exotic, complex pieces. Direct-mail and

FIGURE 1

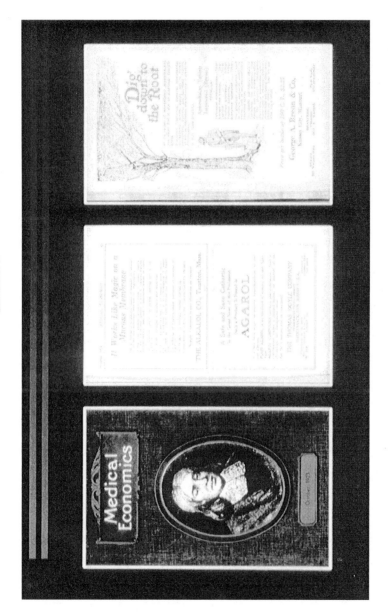

FIGURE 2

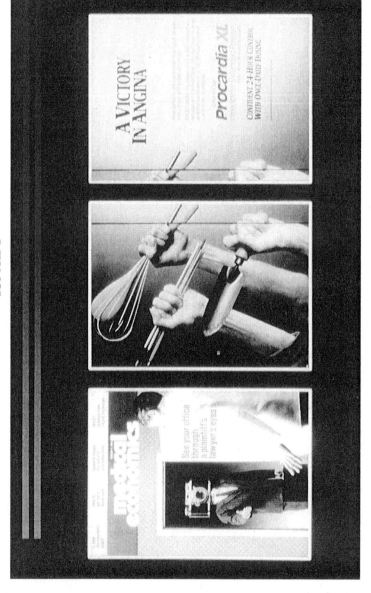

FIGURE 3

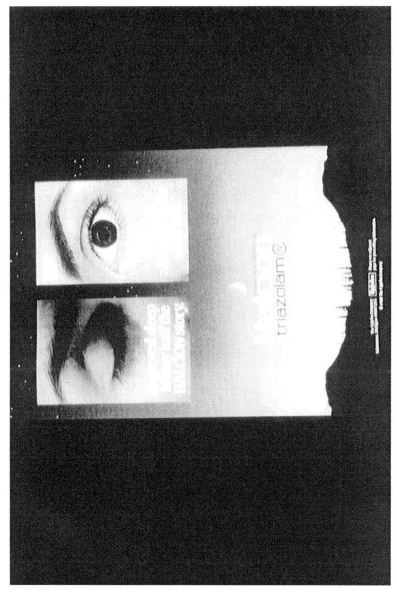

FIGURE 4

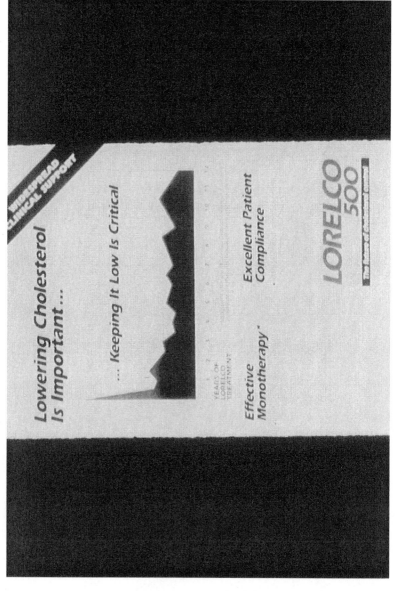

FIGURE 5

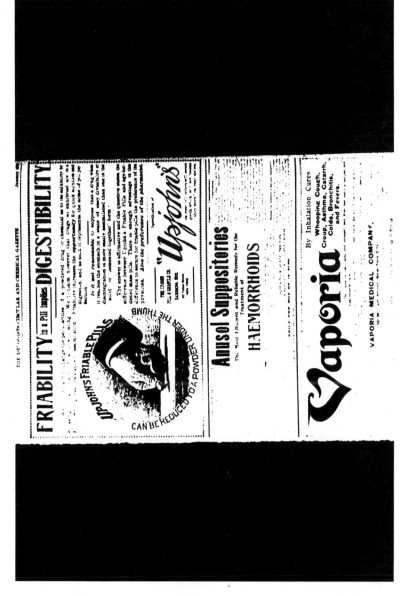

FIGURE 6

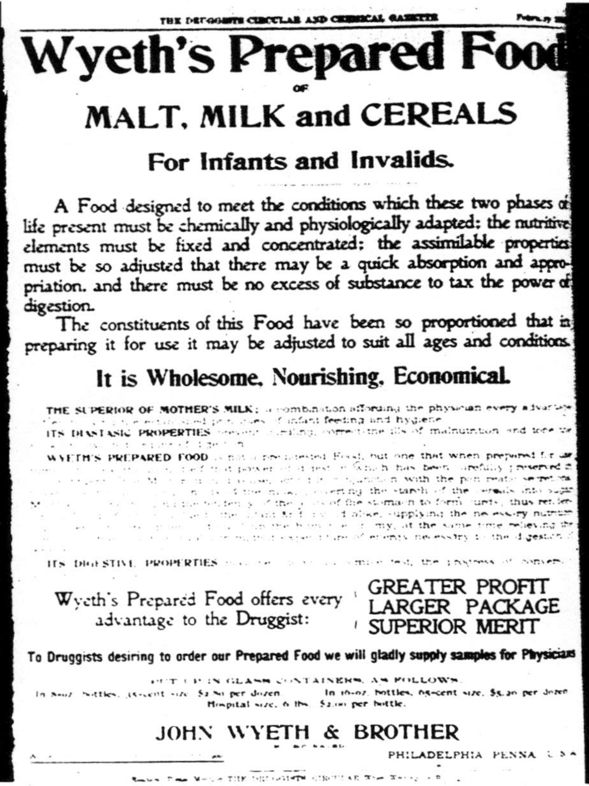
THE DRUGGISTS CIRCULAR AND CHEMICAL GAZETTE

Wyeth's Prepared Food

OF

MALT, MILK and CEREALS

For Infants and Invalids.

A Food designed to meet the conditions which these two phases of life present must be chemically and physiologically adapted: the nutritive elements must be fixed and concentrated; the assimilable properties must be so adjusted that there may be a quick absorption and appropriation, and there must be no excess of substance to tax the power of digestion.

The constituents of this Food have been so proportioned that in preparing it for use it may be adjusted to suit all ages and conditions.

It is Wholesome, Nourishing, Economical.

THE SUPERIOR OF MOTHER'S MILK; a combination affording the physician every advantage ... of infant feeding and hygiene.

ITS DIASTASIC PROPERTIES ... the ills of malnutrition and tone the ...

WYETH'S PREPARED FOOD ... but one that when prepared for use ... has been carefully preserved ... with the pancreatic secretions ... the starch of the cereals into sugar ... of the stomach to form curds, thus render... also, supplying the necessary nutrim... at the same time relieving the ... necessary to the digestion ...

ITS DIGESTIVE PROPERTIES ... the progress of conver...

Wyeth's Prepared Food offers every advantage to the Druggist: GREATER PROFIT / LARGER PACKAGE / SUPERIOR MERIT

To Druggists desiring to order our Prepared Food we will gladly supply samples for Physicians

PUT UP IN GLASS CONTAINERS, AS FOLLOWS.

In 16-oz. bottles, 65-cent size, $5.20 per dozen. Hospital size, 6 lbs. $2.00 per bottle.

JOHN WYETH & BROTHER

PHILADELPHIA PENNA U.S.A.

FIGURE 7

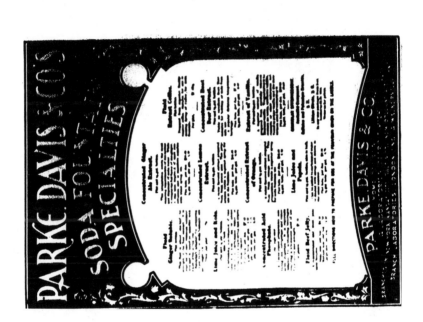

FIGURE 8

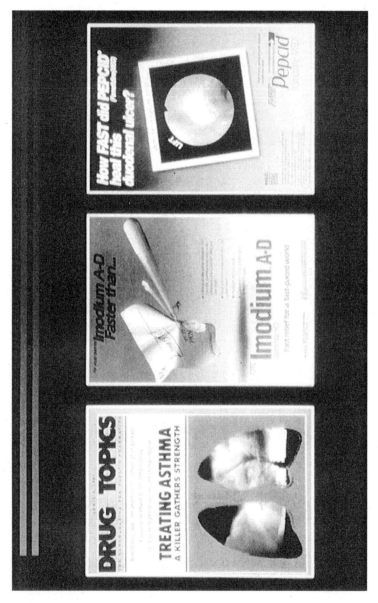

journal advertising complement one another. Journal advertising is designed to attract attention and create awareness of the product. Direct-mail advertising is designed to solicit an immediate response, such as calling an 800 number or completing and mailing a coupon.

We are seeing more direct-mail and journal advertising coming together, with many ads in traditional journals containing 800 numbers, coupons, and business-reply cards. The ability to target a specific audience and the high cost of direct mail, especially skyrocketing postage costs, are major factors. A typical direct-mail package can cost $500 or more to mail 1,000 pieces.

Traditionally, the pharmaceutical industry has relied on the manufacturer's sales representative to get its message across to health care providers. It is estimated that among the major pharmaceutical companies there are anywhere from a few hundred to a few thousand representatives per company. In health care, these representatives call primarily on the physician. However, during the 1990s, we will see the target shift to a larger power base of decision makers. In addition to physicians, this group will include pharmacists, nurses, dentists, benefits managers, insurance companies, and third-party administrators in government and private circles. We must also include health maintenance organizations (HMOs) and other managed care systems. Some see the pharmaceutical companies handling the sales situation by the formulation of sales teams, with each member having an important role: one member for consumer knowledge, one for product knowledge, and one for use and application of the product.

In pharmaceutical promotion, we will clearly see the development of a number of new and innovative ways to advertise and promote products during the next five years. Pharmaceutical companies will be investing in new technologies and strategies to make their audiences aware of product features. More attention will be focused on drug benefits and controlling costs through pharmacy and therapeutics committees, drug formularies, and drug utilization review.

It is estimated that more than one-half of new prescription sales will be directly influenced by private and government third-party programs by the year 2000. Figure 9 displays a type of advertising you will be seeing; these ads were published in *Business and Health*. This magazine is circulated to executives of corporations who have decision-making responsibilities for employee health care plans. The readership also includes top executives of insurance companies, HMOs, and hospitals.

Notice that these ads are not product oriented. There are no multipage announcements of a new beta blocker or H_2 antagonist. Rather, the chief financial officer of XYZ Corporation, for example, is advised that Up-

FIGURE 9

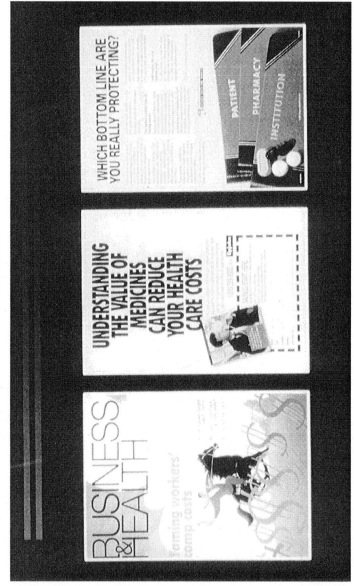

16

john and Marion Merrell Dow Products are designed to complement XYZ's health care and management programs with regard to cost-effectiveness, educational support, and total value. In other words, the brand-name pharmaceutical manufacturers want to shift the focus away from acquisition price to what they see as long-term value. The general message is that branded pharmaceuticals have value, too; the specific message is that mandatory generic substitution and closed formularies do not necessarily provide long-term value.

Now let's shift to an area that has been of deep concern to many marketers and, I am sure, to the FDA: direct-to-consumer advertising. It was not many years ago that pharmaceutical companies would not even think of advertising prescription drugs directly to the consumer. But in today's competitive marketplace, more and more companies are promoting their products in consumer media as well as continuing their ads in medical and professional journals. We have all seen ads to the consumer on Rogaine®, Robitussin®, Nicorette®, and Procardia®. Some feel that in a few years prescription drug ads to consumers will become as commonplace as over-the-counter (OTC) product advertising. Remember when Sandoz ran an ad in 25 major U.S. newspapers promoting its antihistamine Tavist® to doctors reading their local press? That pioneering effort did not take place too long ago–1987. The FDA asked Sandoz to halt the ad because some questions were raised on the product, not because the ad was directed to consumers.

The increase in consumer advertising of prescription products is hampered in part by what it costs to advertise. For example, the full disclosure information, many times, takes a whole page of advertising in fine print; a TV commercial could take about five minutes of air time to divulge all of the product information. The rules for disclosure information were regulated first as a result of the Kefauver Committee's work in 1959. More recently, the FDA ruled that any consumer-oriented ad for a brand-name ethical drug must include all of the information that is in the package insert for the drug, such as information on contraindications, recommended dosage, and possible side effects. Establishing possible new guidelines is one of the top priorities of our new FDA commissioner.

I believe that manufacturers realize that keeping up consumer advertising takes a long-term investment of significant dollars. Of note, however, is that we are hearing that doctors are increasingly willing to prescribe drugs that their patients request. Also, consumers are being made more aware of products and treatments for their problems, and this encourages them to visit their doctor. Case studies at Johns Hopkins Medical School showed that doctors see educated patients as troublesome, but give them better care. Let us keep in mind that in the case of prescription products and former prescription drugs that are now OTC, professionals must be made aware of the medical nature of the products before and during the consumer campaigns. Consumers who are driven by advertising will most often seek the advice of medical professionals, asking if the product is good for themselves and their families. At this critical point, medical professionals hold the success of the product in their hands. As someone said to me recently, millions of dollars' worth of TV or print advertising to consumers cannot do what a pharmacist or physician can accomplish in one day.

Another example of the health care professional's influence came out of a survey *Drug Topics* conducted on pharmacists and patient relations. The data confirmed that the consumer continues to seek out the pharmacist for over-the-counter drug recommendations. Four out of five times, the average pharmacist recommends specific brand-name products to consumers, and 87% of the time, the consumer purchases the brand recommended by the pharmacist. Product compliance has to be at least as high when a brand is recommended by a physician.

Advertising is of assistance to the consumer in making product choices. The OTC product shelf display that is often seen by the consumer in a typical drugstore can create confusion. Because of the numerous choices offered and the competitiveness of the brands, the consumer can be confused about product selection. Advertising helps the consumer make a choice. Advertising to health care professionals provides them with information on product difference, ingredients, side effects, and dosage, all of which aid in the recommendation and choice of a product.

As we said before, direct-to-consumer advertising is on the rise. And, interestingly, physicians and pharmacists feel that, in many cases, such advertising helps them in dealing with the patient. Physicians are discovering that direct-to-consumer pharmaceutical advertising can encourage patients to visit their offices, creating new economic opportunities. Dr. Robert Portman, Chairman of the Woodbridge Group in Woodbridge, New Jersey, made this comment: "Direct-to-consumer medical advertising is here to stay, and why not?" Dr. Portman continues,

> Finally, the consumer has the opportunity to learn about the medication his physician prescribes, including any of its side effects. Today's health-conscious consumer will not go back to the "good old days" when he had no alternative but to accept the purported omniscience of his physician. Let the consumer/patient have his say, let him ask his questions, and let him expect to have those

questions answered to his satisfaction. Why do Senator Kennedy and Congressman Dingell wish to regulate what we hear? Why minimize the amount of information available to us on issues concerning our own health?

The pharmacist's role is also changing in the present environment. He/She is being encouraged to move closer, up front, in the workstation to encourage conversation with the patient. For years, the pharmacist's role was just in the preparation of the drug product, with the transfer of drug information being the responsibility of the physician. Today, the pharmacist is recognized as the expert for drug information and is involved in selecting drugs, monitoring their use, and counseling the patient. There are an estimated 175,000 active pharmacists, and two-thirds work in community settings. According to a *Drug Topics* survey, each pharmacist can have a minimum of 3,000 drug discussions a year with customers. This works out mathematically to 346 million drug discussions by the retail pharmacy community with the consumer. The pharmacist in both independent and chain store environments is encouraged to talk with the consumer or, to put it more professionally, offer patient counseling.

Again, to confirm the growing interest of the consumer in health matters, the *PDR*, which all of us use as a reference source, has become a major seller in bookstores across the country in the nonfiction category. In 1986 it was Number 1. Armed with this information, the consumer is better informed about pharmaceutical products, but he or she will continue to ask the pharmacists, dentists, or doctors for their professional opinions.

Let's look where we are headed. In advertising, as in other businesses, technology is transforming choice, and choice is transforming the marketplace. We will be witnessing new marketing and advertising strategies. One new strategy is the emergence of the so-called nontraditional media. Here we include such vehicles as video, cable TV, radio, audio tapes, seminars and conferences, and symposia. On symposia alone, more than $85 million is spent; 15 years ago spending was only $5 million. Then there are supplements and advertorials; cooperative mailings; pricing guides; and desktop media such as prescription pads, calendars, and appointment books. Again, all of these items are intended to create interest and to inform the targeted audience about a product. Manufacturers continue trying to measure their return on investment in advertising. Here, as elsewhere, this is a difficult thing to do because of the many intangibles involved in advertising.

In the nontraditional area, we are going to see a lot more video broadcasting via satellite during the next few years. I understand that there is a cardboard videocassette ready to be introduced into the market that will play seven times and self-destruct. These technologies will reduce cost significantly. We should also see more automated or electronic voice responses; this is a technique that marries a computer to a telephone keypad, adding a new dimension to telemarketing.

The flowchart shown in Figure 10 illustrates the synergy that exists within the different methods of advertising. Sponsored by Merck, this program–called a *Feeling Fine Program*–used automated voice response to enroll physicians in the AMA's massive campaign against cholesterol. Doctors were made aware through journal ads and direct mail that they could receive a cholesterol screening kit by sending back a business-reply card or calling an 800 number. About 80% of the physicians who enrolled by telephone used a preassigned number to identify themselves, saving a great deal of transcription time and reducing the potential for errors that occur when callers identify themselves verbally. This is an example of synergy within electronics and advertising.

Knowledge of new products will continue to be critical. Between 1985 and 1989, the number of new drugstore products grew by 60%. Fast technologies will aid in the distribution of this information. One way, of course, is the computer. It is astounding to hear that 20 years ago there were only 50,000 computers in use; today more than 50,000 computers are purchased each day.

Successful companies are adapting product to fit customer needs. In the past, companies focused more on changing customers' minds to fit the product. There will be more customer involvement in the product. The manufacturer will communicate and share his product knowledge by better defining the way his company does business, thus gaining credibility.

Marketing a product will depend upon services offered. For example, a large corner drugstore may stock thousands of products, from cosmetics to aspirin. Those products are for sale, but the store is really marketing a service: the convenience of having so much variety in one location.

There is talk of marketing workstations. These stations will draw on graphics, video, audio, and other research information from a variety of databases. From the workstation, the marketer will be able to create and test advertisements, evaluate media options, and analyze viewer and readership data. Marketers will be able to obtain instant feedback on concepts and plans. Thus, the consumer will be both designer and consumer of a product.

These are just a few of the new concepts on the horizon. Many others will be coming. As we move into the twenty-first century, advertising

FIGURE 10

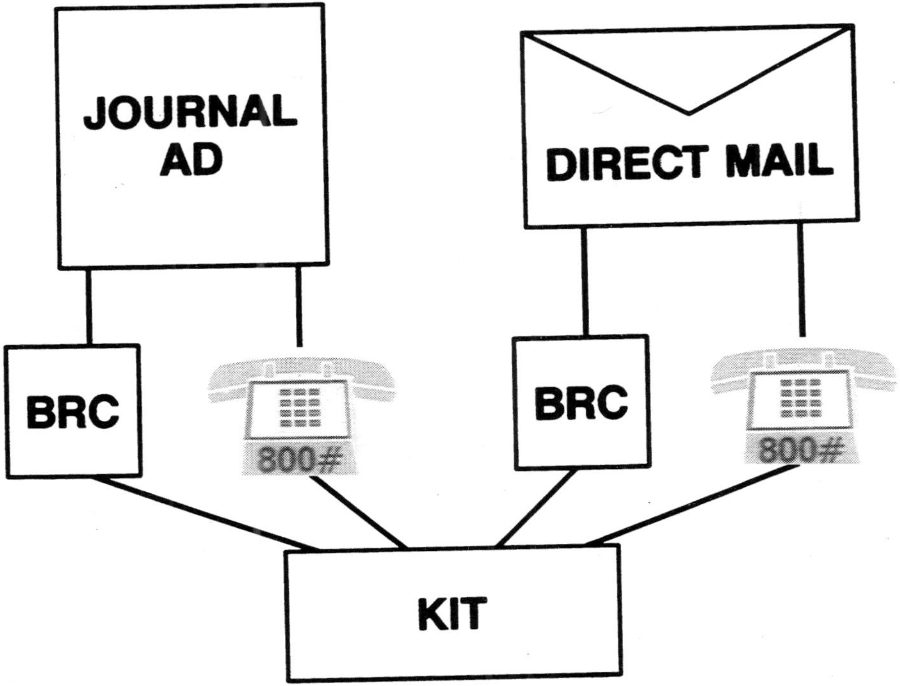

DIRECT MAIL

800#

BRC

JOURNAL AD

800#

BRC

KIT

will be as important as it is now to communicate the vast amount of knowledge that is associated with a product and its application. Only the format of advertising will change, and you and I, hopefully, will continue to welcome it as an integral part of our lives.

Medical Marketing Communications Today: Use and Abuse

Martin E. Cearnal

Medical marketing communication is much more than advertising. Communication takes place in a number of ways, and the entire process–especially as it applies to health care products–is focused on fostering the *appropriate* use of a pharmaceutical product. Any other use of that product can result in problems at all levels.

COMMUNICATION TRENDS

The free-world market for pharmaceutical products is estimated to be approximately $170 billion, depending on which products, categories, and price levels are used. The share of that market in the United States is about 30%, which translates to about $50 billion. The communication activities used to maintain or increase these sales are roughly 8% to 9% of the sales level, or about $4.5 billion. Approximately $3.1 billion is spent on sales forces and the literature and samples those sales forces distribute. Advertising and direct-mail spending is about $700 million, and the use of medical education is about $400 million. Other forms of media and communication amount to approximately $300 million annually.

It is important to recognize that we are seeing a significant rise in the diversity of media and increasing use of educational approaches. In the 1950s and 1960s, pharmaceutical communication essentially was com-

Martin E. Cearnal is President of Physicians World Communications Group, 400 Plaza Drive, P.O. Box 1505, Seacaucus, NJ 07096.

23

prised of three basic media: sales force, medical journals, and direct mail. But with increasing competition, these media have expanded in virtually every direction for delivery of a message. Thus, almost any form of communication today is a potential means of delivering pharmaceutical information and education.

What are the forces stimulating this diversity? In the halcyon days of pharmaceutical marketing in the 1960s and early 1970s, the level of competition was lower, managed care was a minor factor in the marketplace, and most U.S. pharmaceutical products were being sold by the companies that invented them. The level of cross-licensing was much lower, patent protection was longer, and the generic segment was weak. In the last 20 years, all of these factors have changed in ways that make it more difficult to secure adequate return on the cost of bringing a new pharmaceutical product to the market. Recouping the research and development investment requires strategies that achieve the maximum appropriate sales level for a product in the shortest amount of time.

Diffusion of innovation in one form or another is used by most marketers today to deal with this problem. The theory and testing of the diffusion on innovation concept was developed in the 1950s at the University of Iowa. Research demonstrating its validity was completed using agricultural products. This method for organizing communication has repeatedly shown that delivering the right messages in the right order to the right audiences can accelerate the rate at which new concepts are accepted.

Today, companies employ this diffusion of innovation theory through the use of more advisory board activities, symposia, and video conferences, as well as by more effective use of disseminated clinical investigations. All of these techniques provide more extensive information to appropriate audiences earlier in the product's life cycle. In this way, information is available to potential users and opinion leaders much earlier than it was in the past.

As these techniques are combined with the more traditional ones, the classic areas of sales and promotion are moving closer to medical education. They are, in fact, beginning to overlap. This is understandable because the world of the 1990s is a much more complicated one. Problems are no longer as simple as whether or not a new tablet is bioavailable. Now, for example, we are trying to understand how the interleukins may interact with other factors in an immunologic disease. The product concepts to be communicated are more complex and require a much greater educational component.

As audiences become more sophisticated, they demand a higher level of information before making a decision. This means that solid, data-based information, organized, prioritized, and integrated, is required to ensure cost-effective communication.

SELECTING THE MEDICAL MESSAGE

Medical marketing communication as promotion is constrained by approved product labeling, medical ethics, and available media. These constraints form a communication box. Often, in solving creativity problems, we talk of getting out of the box. More realistically, perhaps, we move from a smaller box to a larger one. This movement is an important trend in medical marketing communications.

Promotional communication is subject to the labeling constraints mandated by the Food and Drug Administration (FDA). Some companies have found ways to move beyond these constraints by broadening their communication beyond product information. If a pharmaceutical product message formulated to respect FDA requirements can be married to developments in medicine, the success of the product will become synergized. The communication impact is stronger because the message gets aligned with medical trends that are gaining currency. This type of educational communication is good both for medicine and for pharmaceutical products.

An example of this approach is a recently introduced product used in diagnostic radiology. Communication for this product is linked to a trend taking place in diagnostic imaging wherein magnetic resonance imaging (MRI) is replacing computerized tomography (CT) for many indications. Much of the communication surrounding the product is based on increasing the appropriate use of MRI because use of the product will accompany expansion of the procedure.

In this way, *medically relevant communication* harnesses the power of good medicine to enhance product acceptance and to increase sales by focusing on a convergence of three sets of needs: those of the patient, those of the product, and those of the company. Communication around the convergence point can take place honestly and openly because everyone benefits. This communication technique works at every stage of a product's life cycle, as long as good medicine is involved.

WILL MEDICAL EDUCATION INCREASE?

Three recent studies support the position that educational investments will continue to increase. The first is a study, published in 1988, that compared three continuing medical education (CME) courses sponsored by Georgetown University (1). They were underwritten by the industry, but all of them were designed to meet Accreditation Council on Continuing Medical Education (ACCME) guidelines. These guidelines ensure not only that all communication is open and objective, but also that all appropriate product technologies that apply to the disease entity are discussed, regardless of the underwriter. The studied program included an open discussion of competing technologies. Interestingly, the sponsoring companies' products always received greater benefit than competing products. In other words, when open and honest communication takes place, products are assessed on their value. The net result is that good products succeed, in this case, probably because the manufacturer had the confidence to sponsor a CME program in the first place.

The second study involved 30 industry executives who were asked to rate 10 forms of media on the basis of the information and influence they provided (2). They were effectively being polled for the type of communication they would use in the future. The top three media were sales representatives, teleconferences, and symposia. The media that seem to be most effective in communicating more complex messages are coming to the fore.

A large number of studies have looked at physician responses to questions on how they learn, how they acquire information, and what media they feel have the greatest impact on them. The study discussed here is the most recent, performed in March 1991, and comes from the U.K. literature (3). The top four sources of information cited in this study of physicians are:

- Self-training and experience, which includes CME-type education
- Scientific papers
- Colleagues
- Patient preference.

It is particularly interesting that patient preference is becoming an important influence on the British physician in a public health care system just as its importance has grown in the United States in a private system.

ABUSE AND HOW TO AVOID IT

We have already described the pressure to speed the return on investment. Another force that must be recognized is the aspiration of individuals inside pharmaceutical companies to further their careers. They want to succeed, and they want to be seen by their management as contributors to the success of their companies. As a result, they spend time trying to come up with more innovative ways to convey their messages. Sometimes they break ground, presenting information in novel ways. At other times, however, they break the rules, creating abuse in pharmaceutical communication.

The FDA has, for quite some time, focused on six terms in assessing pharmaceutical communication:

- Content-Is it truthful and fairly balanced? For promotion, does it match approved labeling?
- Context-What is the setting? How was the faculty selected?
- Audience-Is it appropriate for the information?
- Medium of Communication-Is it appropriate for the audience?
- Rationale of Communication-Does it have genuine educational merit?
- Intent-Does the pattern of conduct demonstrate commitment to objective communication?

Case 1

In January 1988, data on an unapproved indication for an approved product was published in the *Journal of the American Medical Association* (4). Publication of the material was, of course, legitimate. The problem occurred when the manufacturer supported a press conference, produced press release materials, and sponsored a luncheon at which the researcher discussed his study. At this point, the FDA cried, "Foul!" While the researcher was at liberty to do anything he wanted with his data, the company was, in the eyes of the FDA, guilty of trying to circumvent regulations that control the communication of an unapproved indication. In this case, the FDA reacted rather quickly because the forum was a press conference. Had the communication been restricted to a small group of experts, the FDA probably would have had no concern.

Case 2

A journal supplement sponsored by a single manufacturer reported results of an open, uncontrolled study of a nitroglycerin patch (5). The results communicated by the manufacturer indicated that the patch was superior to its main competing product, oral isosorbide dinitrate, in reducing anginal attacks. The FDA reacted based on a large, recently completed, well-controlled study in which the company also participated and which had shown an opposite result. As the company began very aggressively to promote the results of the uncontrolled study rather than the controlled study, the FDA reacted. It thought that the company had violated FDA principles in terms of content, context, rationale, and intent.

Case 3

A benzodiazepine manufacturer has, since 1987, been supporting an educational program that is operated under the auspices of an independent advisory board. The board established the educational needs through a validated assessment process, set learning objectives for the program, guided the development of the program content, set the steps of implementation, secured accreditation, and conducted evaluations on every event in the program series. The program has included symposia, videotapes, publications, and teaching materials–including those published by the American Psychiatric Press–and has reached more than 100,000 physicians. Additionally, the program is reaching a rapidly growing number of pharmacists. The program consistently receives commendation, and sales of the supporting manufacturer's product have increased. Although the product has been in the marketplace for four years, the attention paid to objective development and implementation has resulted in no FDA action.

In the future, more and more companies will succeed in using educational communication. Some mistakes have been and will be made during the learning process; other mistakes will be made because of overzealousness. As the industry matures and increases self-regulation, new skills will help companies elect what to do and what to support.

EVOLVING GUIDELINES

The ground rules for CME are established by the ACCME, which will continue to establish the educational standards for all CME providers and organizers.

The American Medical Association (AMA) approaches education from a different point of view–that of physician ethics and ethical communication practices. The AMA was concerned because of the increasing use of various kinds of incentives to encourage physicians to attend meetings or to participate in programs. As a result, a very stringent set of AMA guidelines has been instituted.

The FDA speaks for government and to pharmaceutical companies–sometimes politely, sometimes rather harshly–about the process of new drug approval, regulations, labeling, and, of course, compliance and accuracy of communications.

One of the many roles of the Pharmaceutical Manufacturers Association (PMA) is to speak for industry to the individual company members in areas of policy-making, marketing, and promotion. The guidelines that will govern future communications, medical education, advertising, and promotional activities were adopted by the AMA on 4 December 1990 and by the PMA, in an almost identical form, three days later.

Highlights from AMA/PMA Guidelines

Gifts to physicians from industry that are considered acceptable are those:

- Of modest value and of benefit to the patient
- Related to the physician's work (e.g., pens, pencils)
- Used to underwrite medical conferences (which are seen as beneficial)
- Social events and modest meals that are part of an overall program.

Considered unacceptable are:

- Cash payments to physicians
- Extravagant gifts, even those of patient benefit
- Gifts with strings attached
- Reimbursement for travel, lodging, personal expenses, or time.

Faculty may accept honoraria and reimbursement for expenses incurred through conferences. Consultants, if, in fact, they have consulted, may receive reasonable compensation. Token consulting is not a suitable justification for compensation for travel, lodging, time, etc. Payments to defray cost should not go directly from the company to the physician.

Highlights from the ACCME Guidelines

The conduct of CME meetings should be as recommended by the ACCME guidelines. An accredited sponsor is not a pharmaceutical company but, rather, a university, medical school, or hospital, someone whom the ACCME has accredited to organize CME programs. In ACCME terminology, the person who provides the money is called a grantor, not a sponsor. The control of content, faculty, and material, therefore, belongs to the accredited sponsor in ACCME guidelines. Presentations must be balanced to include all therapeutic options and financial support. Any grantor must be acknowledged in print, without the mention of a specific product.

IMPLICATIONS AND REACTIONS

These changes and guidelines have important implications for communicators and marketers. At a time of changing regulations, companies need to look at new policies, and for policies to be effective across an entire company, senior management must be involved. There is increasing need for self-regulation, without which physician or competitor complaints will stimulate further regulation by the FDA.

Recently, a letter appeared in the *Journal of the American Medical Association*, signed by Dr. Marvin Moser, a leading expert in the field of hypertension, and 12 other hypertension specialists (6). They were responding to a series of seminars and press conferences in which data had been reported that they believed distorted the information available on the treatment of high blood pressure. The authors write, "If we are to continue to practice medicine based on scientific data and not industry sponsored promotional medical education programs and/or public relations inspired media efforts, we must take a stand against unscientific prescribing pressure." It is important for the industry to recognize that physicians are their allies and that constructing programs that generate this kind of response is not in anyone's best interest.

The world of medical marketing communications today is not getting easier. Of the many difficult choices that lie ahead, a major one is whether to consult or to confront the FDA. In a recent speech, David Banks said,

> Many, both inside and outside the Food and Drug Administration, believe that the agency has allowed firms to get away with too much, and the price to be paid by the industry for instances of promotional abuse has not been great enough. Perhaps the only means for the agency to gain many firms' attention is with the regulatory equivalent of a body slam. (7)

The range of responses available to the FDA has been inadequate. New powers of enforcement probably will include a broader range of tactics to control inappropriate activities by pharmaceutical companies.

How should the industry respond to this? One way is with an industry-wide initiative to self-regulate with the objective of establishing a new level of trust between industry and the FDA.

A WORD ABOUT PATIENT INTERESTS

Much discussion has been given to the drug lag in the United States. An example of this is a drug currently pending at the FDA that has been approved in 39 countries. Every major Western European country has approved it. Recently, it was approved for over-the-counter sale in Canada. But it is not available in the United States, even by prescription. The United States does have a primary drug lag, in part due to the shortage of resources at the FDA and in part to application of those resources. It is, however, only the first drug lag.

An information lag is developing as the rate of innovation increases. This information lag causes pharmaceutical companies to deliver yesterday's message with today's medication. The problem develops when an innovative physician or medical center discovers that an unapproved use of an approved product confers a significant patient benefit. The regulations dictate that the pharmaceutical company must submit well-controlled studies to the FDA and receive approval before communicating this information. Pursuing the approval requires a major shift in resource allocation by the company. Additionally, the FDA has finite resources with which to review information, so when the new information arrives, it falls in line waiting to be processed. The resulting dilemma is that companies cannot communicate important information about their already-approved products, even if the information may save lives. This problem needs special attention. Because of this lag, companies are conveying product information that medical experts consider outdated, but the FDA has not received adequate information to grant approval for new claims and therefore sees significant potential risks.

Solutions may exist, but they are never easy. The appropriate objective is to improve patient care through the timely communication of valid information. This requires a series of steps. First, the industry should propose guidelines for communication in this area. Next, the FDA should review, modify, and eventually approve the guidelines and establish appropriate measurement criteria. Adding independent editorial control of the content of communications to the six criteria historically endorsed by the FDA could be a basis for starting these discussions. Until the guidelines are refined, this remains an important problem. Consultation between the companies and the FDA is the only strategy to pave the way for improved patient care in this area.

CONCLUSION

Medical marketing communication fills a critical need in the process of enhancing health care. Although commercial pressures and oversights cause occasional abuses, the vast majority of communication meets all legal and ethical constraints and standards. The increasing complexity of medical information is leading to increased use of education as a communication tool. Education that links product information to developing medical trends can enhance the quality of patient care and product acceptance while complying with FDA regulations, AMA/PMA/ACCME guidelines, and the tenets of sound medical practice.

REFERENCES

1. Bowman MA, Pearle DL. Changes in drug prescribing patterns related to commercial company funding of continuing medical education. J Contin Educ Health Prof 1988;8:13-20.

2. Roseman E. Where the changing promotional mix is headed. Med Market Media 1989;(June):10-20.

3. Anon. Effectiveness of UK pharma reps. SCRIP World Pharm News 1991;1596:4.

4. Weiss JS, Ellis CN, Headington JT, Tincoff T, Hamilton TA, Voorhees JJ. Topical tretinoin improves photoaged skin: a double-blind vehicle-controlled study. JAMA 1988;259:527-32.

5. Anon. Angina pectoris: treatment update. Intern Med World Rep 1989;(May Supp).

6. Moser M, Blaufox MD, Freis E, et al. Who really determines your patients' prescriptions? JAMA 1991;265:498-500.

7. Banks D. Unpublished.

Prescription Drug Advertising: An Industry Perspective

Peter R. Seaver

When we talk about promotion, it is a good idea to make certain we are talking about the same thing. For instance, imagine you own a circus. If you paint a sign that says, "Circus coming to the fairgrounds Saturday" and give the grocer two free tickets to put the sign in his window, that's ADVERTISING. If you put the sign on the back of an elephant and parade it through town, that's PROMOTION. And if the elephant walks through the mayor's flower garden, that's PUBLICITY. But if you can get the mayor to laugh about it, that's PUBLIC RELATIONS. For the purpose of this paper, I will narrow my focus to advertising. I will use a commonly accepted definition: "Advertising is a controlled commercial message appearing in purchased time or space."

Advertising and other forms of pharmaceutical promotion have come under intense scrutiny. But I want you to know that I am proud that The Upjohn Company is an advertiser. I am proud of our advertising: *proud* of the talented people who create it, *proud* of the quality products we advertise, and *proud* that these products benefit millions of people in more than 150 countries worldwide. Therefore, we take the responsibility of advertising our products very seriously.

I want to impress upon you six basic points:

- First, advertising pharmaceuticals is a complex undertaking because of the nature of our products, our markets, and our customers.
- Second, we realize that there is much to learn about pharmaceutical advertising, and we continually work to perfect our craft.
- Third, advertising is designed to leverage the efforts of a company's sales force.

Peter R. Seaver is Corporate Vice President for Worldwide Marketing, The Upjohn Company, 7000 Portage Road, Kalamazoo, MI 49001.

- Fourth, pharmaceutical advertising contributes not only to my livelihood, but to yours as well.
- Fifth, the sales generated by advertising today enable research-based companies to discover and develop the drugs of tomorrow.
- And sixth, prescription product advertising improves the practice of medicine and by so doing improves the lives of millions of patients.

Here is an interesting quiz to get us started. Who said: "Advertisements contain the only truths to be relied upon in newspapers"? How many of you said William Randolph Hearst? How about Will Rogers? Or our good friend Ken Feather? Well, the answer is Thomas Jefferson. It is impossible to know whether Jefferson made that statement out of frustration with inaccurate news stories or assumed advertisers had better tell the truth or they would be out of business. I like to believe that Jefferson was giving advertisers the benefit of the doubt.

I suspect some of you think differently: that truths *are* stretched, that claims *are* made that cannot be substantiated, and that flights of fancy not only appear on the editorial pages of our newspapers and magazines, but frequently in advertisements as well. But when people criticize advertising, I suspect they define it differently than those who practice it. In 1904, Albert Lasker, the father of the profession, defined advertising as "salesmanship in print." While advertising is more sophisticated today and extends far beyond print media, that definition still holds true.

Let me tell you a brief but relevant story about Albert Lasker, who worked for and later bought the Lord and Thomas advertising agency in Chicago in the early part of the twentieth century. At that time, agencies only sold space in magazines and newspapers. They did not create advertising as we know it. There were no creative advertising departments. Back then, agencies were solely concerned with placing ads to remind consumers of a product and the product's intended use.

Lasker, however, recognized the potential of advertising to inform and persuade. He set about creating a new genre of print advertisements for Lord and Thomas. His genius amassed him great wealth, so much so that he sold the agency in 1940 and devoted the rest of his life to philanthropy. Lasker founded the Albert and Mary Lasker Foundation for Research of Heart Disease, Cancer, and Mental Illness. The annual Lasker Foundation Award is recognized as one of the most prestigious honors bestowed in medicine throughout the world. Ten recipients have been Nobel laureates. How wonderfully satisfying it is to realize that a good portion of the fortune Lasker built from creative advertising was dedicated to improving the practice of medicine in the United States.

Over time, advertising has evolved to the point where the American economic system cannot function without it. That bears repeating for the devotees of public radio and public television: there is absolutely no way that the American economic system can function without advertising. But some of you might be thinking: "But oh, how much more pleasant it would be." While we might associate advertising with loud car salesmen in loud suits, we should also recognize its positive influence on economic growth and public health in America.

Think about margarine and the advertisements that led millions of people to switch from butter to margarine. This wasn't the federal government attempting to change people's eating habits, but an opportunity for private enterprise to sell low-fat, polyunsaturated products. And consider the revolution that occurred in dental hygiene. How much of the daily brushing would be going on now if we had not had 50 years of tasteful and effective advertising on behalf of toothpaste? Toothpaste improves your breath, helps remove tartar, and provides fluoride to prevent cavities.

You may have heard about a recent study documenting the power of advertising to change health habits. The study assessed the impact of a single commercial directed at men who risked contracting colon cancer. As a result of viewing the television commercial, the number of men who consulted their physicians about colon cancer more than doubled in the four test markets. The Advertising Research Foundation projected that if this single-commercial campaign had been broadcast throughout the country, it would have persuaded 2.7 million men over the age of 40 to consult their physicians about the disease.

In a similar vein, pharmaceutical advertising has positively influenced the medical community by informing them of new drugs, new indications, and new formulations. As a result, the medical publishing industry has thrived, and medical journals continue to be the physician's primary source of up-to-date information.

It is important to appreciate the complexity of advertising prescription pharmaceuticals, where companies must consider myriad questions involving the product, the market, the customers, and the Food and Drug Administration (FDA). Let me share some of the questions we ask ourselves as we go about the task of creating advertising. Where is the product in its life cycle? Is it new? Is it unknown by name or mode of action to the prescribing community? Or is it a mature product, a product that has an established place in the practice of medicine, one that requires ads that remind, sustain, nurture, and reinforce previous prescribing decisions? Or, on the other hand, is the product indeed in the final stages of its life cycle, losing market because its patent has expired or newer, better products are available? Such products may, nevertheless, warrant advertising because they remain the preferred treatment option of a devoted group of prescribers. Examples of such established products are Provera® and Premarin®.

Another question is: What are the characteristics of the market? Is the market satisfied or dissatisfied with current products? An example of an unsatisfied market is nonsteroidals. Physicians often switch back and forth among the dozen or so nonsteroidal drugs in search of one that works for a particular patient. On the other hand, some segments of the antibiotic market are quite satisfied, as physicians prescribe one or two drugs that knock out an infection very effectively in nearly all patients. There are other market characteristics to consider as well. Is the market crowded, such as the market for nonsteroidals? Or, do we need to create a market? Such was the situation for prescription hair growth products before The Upjohn Company introduced Rogaine® in 1989.

Another question we might ask ourselves is whether advertising is required to maintain market share or to increase market share. The answer helps determine how much to spend. If you gain approval for a new indication for a well-established product, your advertising campaign will build upon the foundation that already exists, costing much less than launching a brand-new product.

Here's another question: Is it important in the particular market to inform the target audience about some of the technical aspects of the product, or is it merely enough to remind them why they chose the product in the first place? A product's life-cycle position will help answer this question.

Probably the most important mission we have as advertisers is to create brand-name awareness. It's essential that we achieve ad recognition and tie that recognition to the product name. Advertising enables us to make that connection.

In today's crowded and very noisy marketplace of medicines and medical devices, there is a misconception that a truly important breakthrough product sells itself, that it does not need to be advertised. This just isn't so. Even with favorable coverage in professional journals and word-of-mouth recommendations, new products cannot achieve their true potential without advertising. It does not matter that the product is truly a blockbuster breakthrough or a modification of an existing compound. For research-based companies to recoup their enormous research and development investment, advertising is essential to achieving rapid product momentum and securing a competitive share of the market. What you do in those first six months–some say the first six weeks–will set the angle of the sales curve for the life of that product. After all, a new product is new only once.

Let me digress to discuss direct-to-consumer advertising of prescription pharmaceuticals. Upjohn has figured prominently in this area the past two years because of its various Rogaine campaigns. It has also become a front-burner issue at the FDA, so I think it is important that I share The Upjohn Company's philosophy about direct-to-consumer advertising and why such advertising is appropriate for Rogaine.

Back in 1984, when Upjohn hosted a symposium on the subject, we took the position that consumer advertising should not interfere with the traditional physician-patient relationship. We still believe this. We continue to need physicians–as the informed intermediaries–to help patients make informed drug therapy decisions. However, we also recognize that consumer advertising of *selected products* is appropriate, as long as the physician's role is not compromised and the FDA guidelines are strictly followed.

What types of products or market conditions warrant direct-to-consumer advertising? Until Rogaine, there was no scientifically proven treatment for baldness, until Seldane®, no nonsedating antihistamines, until Nicorette® chewing gum, no prescription substitute for nicotine. Now that these products are available and advertised to the public, patients are seeking their doctor's council and advice in ever-increasing numbers.

With Rogaine, we knew a doctor would not tell his patient: ''I've got good news and bad news. The good news is that your blood pressure is fine and cholesterol is normal. The bad news is that you're going bald and should do something about it.'' I am being facetious, of course, but it became quite clear from the outset that prospective Rogaine patients would have to initiate discussion about their hair loss. In the physician's eyes, hair loss is not a medical problem.

Direct-to-consumer advertising makes sense because consumers are more aware, more educated, more sophisticated about health care than at any other time in history. Advertising can help consumers make informed choices about medicines and alert them to earlier detection of disease.

I understand that the new Commissioner of the Food and Drug Administration, David Kessler, is skeptical about direct-to-consumer advertising, as well as other types of pharmaceutical promotion. If companies *are* violating federal regulations, the FDA is correct to bring them into line. In the process, however, I hope that the FDA does not restrict the activities of companies that have acted correctly and have worked in good faith with the agency.

It should be clear that consumer advertising will never replace advertising to physicians, and pharmaceutical companies will continue to spend a great deal of time and money to reach this informed audience. Physicians spend an estimated 8.6 hours each month reading medical journals, so it is critical that we choose correctly from among the 630 or so medical journals those most likely to be read by the physicians we target. We make those decisions through the use of a sophisticated computer media model. Data from the on-line system enable us to attain optimum reach and frequency for our ads. The really good journals are the ones that the media model recommends and the ones in which we advertise.

This is important because from 1983 to 1988, the size of the industry's sales force increased by 50%. During the same period, the number of office-based physicians grew only 7%. In addition, 20% of office-based physicians no longer see sales representatives, and 30% see a given salesperson less than 3 times per year.

Ninety percent of what research shows to be poor advertising is just that because the product is not correctly positioned in the marketplace, which makes the message neither believable nor relevant. It does not matter if the ad copy is written by Moses with art by Michelangelo if your product is not positioned correctly. How you position your product in the market and against the loyal competition goes a long way toward distinguishing your product. In essence, you must create a theme that is yours alone, one that is believable and relevant. An example from our international business is the theme developed in the 1960s for our antibiotic Lincocin®. The headline–which is still in use today–reads: "Lincocin penetrates, Lincocin works." Four words, two that make the promise and two that reinforce the product name.

Our advertising budgets are developed using a model incorporating data provided by the media model and other inputs from product management. The process begins by establishing goals. We then determine how much money we need to spend to reach these goals. This task-oriented approach to spending has proven more efficient and cost-effective than setting advertising budgets based on percentage of sales.

So, how much should you spend? We have found that each therapeutic category requires a different threshold of advertising exposure before an ad can register an effect on the prescribers. For nonsteroidals for rheumatoid and osteoarthritis, the investment is considerable. Why? In the case of nonsteroidals, there are many products from which to choose, and the target audience is the largest in the industry, including general practitioners, family practitioners, internists, osteopaths, and orthopedic surgeons.

Let's say that the audience has been identified, the communication objectives are carefully laid out, and the advertisement is consistent with the product positioning statement. Now we take the proposed advertisement and ask ourselves three questions that help us to measure and evaluate our work.

First, is the communication clear? Ambiguity spells death for an ad campaign. So, first be clear in your communication. And, surprisingly, despite all the creative talent in the industry, advertising messages sometimes become garbled.

The second question is more specific to the medical side and vital to the pharmaceutical industry: Is it true? Some might say, "Ah, but we have watchdog agencies to make sure that it is indeed true." But I find that professionals are the most likely people to question the claims of our products.

The third question, and one that prompts the most criticism of pharmaceutical advertising is: Is the message believable and relevant to the physician's practice? The message may be as clear as a mountain stream and based on the most fundamental truths since the Ten Commandments. But if the advertising is not believable and relevant, for whatever reason, the product will not achieve its sales potential. Sometimes the truth must be made believable.

Let me give you an example. I am holding one, smaller-than-aspirin-size tablet in my hand. I tell you this tablet is as powerful as injectable morphine in relieving deep, somatic pain. I also tell you that this is a nonnarcotic, nonaddicting substance that can be taken once a day. Indeed, it is a medical breakthrough that was proven in double-blind cross-over studies and brought to you by the finest research-based company in the world.

Now we have created an advertisement that claims that this single tablet is therapeutically equal to multiple injections of morphine for intractable pain. I ask you: Is it believable? If you say no, that your heritage, your fundamental background, refuses to let you believe that, well, I can advertise the product in every prestigious medical journal in the world, but it is still going to be–in your view–an unbelievable claim. Even worse, from our standpoint, is that we would have failed to persuade physicians of our product's value, thereby denying millions of patients of a more effective and humane therapy.

There is another series of questions that we ask ourselves to determine whether our advertising is doing the job for which it was intended. First, is it intrusive? You may be saying to yourself, "I hate to be bothered by ads; I wish they would go away and leave me alone." But the fact is that advertising must have stopping power: it must be noticed. Getting you to refocus your mind on the message is perhaps the essential responsibility of advertising. A lot of good advertising that we see is good because we are stopped but not offended. But you must first be stopped. The advertisement must intrude into your mind and your space.

The second question you have to ask yourself is: Will the ad be read? We attempt to put news into our ads wherever possible, but the key to readership is in the headline. If the headline doesn't have it, the ad doesn't have it. We do tracking studies on our ads to determine how we are communicating with our target audience. In essence, we change our ads when the market tells us to do so.

I have thrown out many questions. I hope they have helped you understand pharmaceutical advertising from an industry perspective. We view pharmaceutical ads as a creative outlet for promoting our products. But I also want to emphasize that, increasingly, we are grounding this art to hard science, which enables us to improve the relevance of our message continually.

I have discussed pharmaceutical advertising up close. Now I would like to take a broader view. You may wonder why I feel so strongly about advertising. It really has to do with what our country is all about. And I am not just focusing on freedom of speech, a logical place to start when you are talking about advertising and the American way. I am taking it to another level. Advertising can and does create huge new prescription markets in this country. As a result, our products have helped save lives, improve lives, and ameliorate disease states of the patients who are our ultimate customers.

In 1957, when the first oral antidiabetic was introduced, insulin was the only way to control blood sugar. The vast majority of patients who were noninsulin dependent but experienced constant hyperglycemia either went untreated or took insulin. Orinase®, you may remember, sat on the pharmacy shelves when it was introduced. (My predecessors at Upjohn remember it very dearly because the product was not meeting the sales forecast.) It was the Upjohn representative-supported by advertising-who, over time, helped to create this new market. Subsequently, Orinase became a hugely successful product, one that brought significant business to pharmacies throughout the country and relief to millions of Type II diabetics.

When aspirin was virtually the only way to relieve the pain and inflammation of arthritis, the market was small and offered few therapeutic alternatives. Patients who could not tolerate the required doses of aspirin suffered horribly. When Motrin® became available, it was The Upjohn Company sales force-together with advertising-that created the market, a market that provided patients relief from their pain, provided income to pharmacists, and rewarded the research-based companies for developing the products. A win-win-win situation.

One of the great medical miracles in the 1970s and 1980s has been the gains made in controlling hypertension. While public education and the work of the National Institutes of Health certainly played a major role in this public health success story, credit should also go to the pharmaceutical industry for creating the market. In recent years, a vast array of new approaches to hypertension created–through advertising–a huge market that did not exist previously.

To compete successfully, research-based companies must have the opportunity to recoup their enormous research investment, which can exceed $230 million for the successful development of a novel entity. Pharmaceutical advertising helps us do that. When done ethically and expertly, advertising is invaluable to the successful marketing of a product. We see it as an essential part of our marketing mix. Indeed, we can make a case that it is the premier support mechanism for the men and women who call upon physicians on behalf of our products.

In the course of these remarks, I hope that you have gained a better understanding for the complexity of advertising prescription pharmaceuticals. I hope, too, that I have convinced you that advertising is essential to communicate to the medical community the availability of new therapies or improvements on established therapies. As long as research-based companies discover, develop, and market new therapies or modify existing therapies, there will be a need for pharmaceutical advertising.

Prescription Drug Advertising:
A Critic's Perspective

Michael R. Waldholz

I often get asked why we do not write more happy news or upbeat news, more promotional news. Recently, I had an interview with a chief executive officer at a top pharmaceutical company who asked me why I had not written about a grant program for scientists that his company so graciously supported every year. It is a nonrestricted grant for scientists in the basic area of cancer research, in immunology and neurology. It involves a lot of money and backs a lot of very important science. I said to him, after he gave his pitch, that I was sure the public ought to know more about it, but I did not want to be so flippant as to tell him to take out an ad. I told him that there was one sure way that I would write about it and that was for him to stop giving out the grant. The story would say how great a program it had been and how terrible it was that the company was no longer giving the grant. He did not think that was very funny. But it's true. Bad news often is what makes news.

I want to preface this paper with the fact that I am a big fan of the pharmaceutical industry. I have been covering it for ten years. Before I came to the *Wall Street Journal*, I really knew nothing about the industry. I came to the *Journal* initially to cover health economics and policy and was put into a slot that also covered the pharmaceutical industry. At the time, I think the editors thought I would pay attention to it with a couple of fingers on my left hand. In fact, the issues that soon arose, such as receptor technology, genetics, biotechnology, competition, the business consolidation that is taking place, and the breakthrough drugs that are coming out based on phenomenal basic research, have really taken up most of my time. I can tell you it is one of the more exciting fields to be covering as a reporter. There are a lot of people at the *Wall Street Jour-*

Michael R. Waldholz is Medical Writer for the *Wall Street Journal*, 200 Liberty Street, New York, NY 10281.

nal who cover a variety of fascinating fields, and I can tell you that I am the envy of many of them. So when I say I am a fan, I am. I think there is a lot that goes on that makes writing and reporting about the pharmaceutical business very exciting. But the industry has not done a good job of communicating that story. Indeed, it has done a number of things that have hurt its reputation, and many of these involve its very aggressive efforts to market its products.

I am reminded of a waking dream I had while at a meeting of an advisory committee for the Food and Drug Administration (FDA). This advisory committee was taking 14 hours to consider an application by Warner-Lambert to market a drug for Alzheimer's disease. The drug is called Cognex®, THA, or tacrine. If approved, it would be the first drug for Alzheimer's, and it was highly controversial. The data for the drug was equivocal, and it was difficult to determine how well it worked, if at all. After 14 hours, I had to do something to keep myself awake. I came up with what I thought would be a great direct-to-consumer ad. The scene takes place in the bedroom of a family. The shades are drawn, the room is darkened, and an elderly woman is sitting on the edge of her bed, complaining to her son that she cannot find her shoes. She cannot remember where they are. This happens to her every day, and she is very angry. Finally, she gets on her shoes. The son walks out of the room and shakes his head. He is met by his wife in the hallway, and she says, "I wish there was something we could do." A voiceover says, "There is. You can see your doctor. Call 1-800-Cognex."

Now why do I say that? It seems to me that in many ways this drug is similar to Rogaine®, a hair growth drug advertised heavily to the public. The Rogaine ad is not the only consumer drug commercial. And it is not going to be the only one that we are going to see in the future. I would be surprised, to be perfectly honest, if, in fact, we do not see an ad something like the Alzheimer's one because this is going to be one of a class of drugs in which the pharmaceutical industry believes the public should be directly contacted.

I am a big fan of advertising. I learn a lot through advertising. I learn that the Camry® is on sale for $12,000, and if I rush to my Tri-State dealer, I can get my $12,000 Toyota Camry. I understand that when I get there, I will probably find out that they either do not have any more $12,000 Camrys or that they just sold the last one. I understand that. I think most Americans are very adept at picking their way through that kind of advertising system. But most of us are not very good at doing that when it comes to medicine. We have a completely different mind-set when it comes to that, and I think that is one of the problems with drug company ads. I think it is going to be very hard for a patient with Alzheimer's disease to make consumer choices similar to those made in buying a car. Still, the trend that we are seeing suggests to me that sometime in the future we are going to see ads like that, and I think it is a real problem.

I have been asked to talk about drug advertising at a meeting that clearly is identified as a discussion of pharmaceutical promotion. But I do not think it would be good for me to limit myself just to advertising; I really want to discuss the whole issue of promotion. I think advertising is just a piece of the puzzle in what the pharmaceutical company does. The industry–with pride–can defend its advertising to doctors, which is highly regulated. But the industry does a lot more promoting than that.

A few years ago, I wrote a story in which I said a certain drug promotion was part of the company's effort to pitch medicine to doctors. Soon after, I got a call from the head of the company's marketing department who said, "We don't pitch medicines, we educate the doctor." I think he was a very sincere fellow, perhaps a lot like many of you, but the point was that he and his company were pitching medicine to doctors and that the word promotion–a nice thing to call what you do–is still marketing. Promotion is sales, and promotion is an innocuous word for the real stuff. There are words with power and meaning like hyping and exaggerating and embellishing and pitching and peddling, pushing, shilling, hawking, hustling, and just plain marketing and sales. You know the pharmaceutical industry is very good at using euphemisms. Marketing conventions are gussied up as scientific symposia where doctors get continuing medical education credit. Salesmen are detailers, and price hikes are justified as recouping research. Free samples are educational materials. Television commercials are public service announcements, and press releases come under the letterhead of consumer interest groups.

You might be saying, "What a cynic." But cover the business side of the pharmaceutical industry as a journalist, and even the sweetest among you will become jaded. I recently walked over to a reporter at the *Wall Street Journal* who covers the airline industry. Now there is an industry with problems. You know it is a largely unregulated industry that thinks nothing of overbooking flights, charging outrageous sums to fly short but little-used routes, losing your luggage, and canceling flights with little or no notice. I asked the reporter for some advice on traveling on a particular airline. He just scowled at me, waved me away, and yelled, "Come on, they are all the same." I figure, well, this guy has had too much time walking that industry beat. But if you walk the pharmaceutical industry beat, you find similar problems.

For instance, I recently received a call from someone at a public relations firm. This was a call from a very nice-sounding woman telling me about an important conference being sponsored by a top medical school on bacterial infections in the aging. Sounds like a great meeting, doesn't it? In fact, after much questioning on my part, I found out that this meeting was sponsored by a pharmaceutical company and involves a drug marketed by McNeil Pharmaceuticals, a Johnson & Johnson unit. Well, fine, now I finally know everything. I am sure it will be a very interesting meeting, and I probably would learn a lot. While I am sure this is going to be a very important meeting, I now feel somewhat duped. No one was hiding anything from me, but it took a little pulling to get a straight answer.

The truth is, maybe I have become a little jaded. I came to the *Wall Street Journal* in June of 1980, and at that time, I was hired to cover the revolution taking place in the economic side of health care, the efforts to control costs, the rise of health maintenance organizations (HMOs) and such. While I did my share of health policy stories, I soon realized that the big story was in the discovery and development of new medicines and in the basic science underlying such efforts. I continue to be excited and amazed by what takes place in the laboratory. I hope my coverage of the biomedical sciences reflects that.

But the business side of the drug industry is a different beast indeed. Soon after I got to the *Journal*, I received a breathless call from a fellow reporter in our Chicago bureau with a story tip. He was certain that this was going to make the front page of the paper once I looked into it. Did I know, he asked, that drug companies take out glitzy and slick advertisements–with full-page graphics and phrases that would make Proctor and Gamble smile–in scientific journals, in magazines that carry science, magazines that doctors read? That was ten years ago, and a lot has happened, including the emergence of such ads directed straight to the public. Few people today could be so breathlessly amazed upon stumbling over such blatant commercialism in medicine. Yet the truth is that, even today, the American public expects something better from its pharmaceutical industry, something different from the kind of marketing we get from General Motors or a liquid detergent maker.

Part of that, of course, is the mystique of the doctor that has emerged since World War II. In those years, doctors were lionized and probably with good reason. But the doctors' fall from grace could have been predicted. Why is that? Well, anyone who develops that kind of power is certain to abuse it, even if it is some small portion of that population. There has been greed, and it has been plenty reported. There has been malpractice, and that has been reported, too. Today doctors are paying a high price for the errors of a few, with more regulation and more skepticism from the public.

Drug makers also rode high before and after World War II. The discovery of penicillin and, later, the polio vaccine is still seen by members of my parents' generation as verging on magic. It was proof that we as a society had entered an age when all things were possible and when men and women in commerce worked for the public good. We as a society had become civilized, and we were above the crass concerns of profit and greed. But then the drug companies themselves made some very highly publicized mistakes. There was the thalidomide problem, then DES, and, more recently, Oraflex® and Zomax®. The industry, just like the doctoring business, developed a tremendous amount of power, took advantage of it, and took it for granted.

Now, I think there are many reasons why the public feels less positive about the drug industry, despite its record of producing important breakthroughs. One reason may be that the only time we really need medicine is when we are sick. And who, of course, are we going to blame when we get sick? We cannot blame ourselves because that would be too painful. Some of us blame God, but some of us cannot. Where can we direct our anger, and who can we blame for at least some small part of our misery: the folks in the medical establishment. At least we can blame them for raising our hopes and then letting us down, for making us think of them as saints and then acting more like the rest of us. It is in this context that we can understand the degree of public dismay. It is outraged and hurt and feels betrayed by an industry that is supposed to be doing God's work. Instead, it winds up doing business with ethics that are sometimes no better–although arguably no worse–than those of the guy at the local car dealership.

I know you have heard this all before, but you know there is a sense that in some ways things are getting worse. In fact, the industry has become more aggressive. The cost of developing drugs is, in fact, rising. I remember when the cost was $80 million and 10 years to produce a drug, and then it jumped to $120 million and 10 years, and before I turned around, it was $230 million. Now I do not dispute that number, but no drug company has ever been willing to open up its books and show me how it spent that money. I know it costs a lot of money to discover new drugs. I have been in the labs. I have seen the kind of expensive machines that have to go in there and the labor-intensive work that is involved. I do not dispute that. But the drug industry has done a very poor job of explaining that side of the story and a very good job of shooting itself in the foot.

Consider that a few years ago there was an effort in Congress to extend Medicare coverage in a variety of areas, and one of those areas would have been to pay for prescription drugs for the elderly. This would have been revolutionary. It is interesting that the pharmaceutical industry was one of the principal lobbyists against that bill and even helped lobby against it once it was passed. Some people in the drug industry were worried that once the government began paying for drugs, it might take advantage of that and begin ratcheting down the prices.

My comments should provide you with some of the reasons why members of Congress are up in arms, regulators are willing to regulate, and the bureaucracy is willing to take a shot at the prescription drug industry, while the public is only getting one side of the message, and many doctors are getting a little concerned. Promotional activity by the pharmaceutical industry has long been the norm. However, in recent years, the amount of money drug companies spend on gifts, reminder items, and especially symposia has escalated sharply. Moreover, the form of the promotion has changed, at times approaching outright bribery. It is quite amazing to me that we have the spectrum of Senate hearings where the American Medical Association makes a statement about a new criteria and guidelines to cover the kinds of gifts that doctors can take. We have to admit that the hearings sponsored by Senator Kennedy have had some impact, otherwise the American Medical Association would not have put out those guidelines, and the pharmaceutical industry would not have provided its endorsement. Indeed, the pharmaceutical industry must be concerned about its image and the amount of money it is spending on drug promotion in the health care community.

All you have to do is read some of the medical journals over the last few years and the printed letters from some disgruntled doctors who have described the kind of deals they have been offered. For instance, one told of a series of fine prints in exchange for allowing the detail person to visit his group more often. Another company sent checks for $156 to senior dermatology residents, supposedly to cover transportation costs to an upcoming American Academy of Dermatology meeting, but really "because . . . we want you to know that we are thinking of you." A third performed free computer research on the topic of the doctor's choice, a service that some doctors used every month to keep abreast of the latest research in their field. A fourth sent groups of doctors, identified particularly as hard sells, on educational weekends of snorkeling in the Caribbean and golfing at Palm Springs and Acapulco.

In fact, such marketing techniques have become commonplace and so disturbing to some that Sidney Wolfe at the Health Research Group has set up a doctor bribery hot line to track industry activities. In his testimony before Senator Kennedy's recent hearings, Dr. Wolfe described numerous ethically shaky drug company schemes reported to him by doctors calling this hot line. For instance, one laboratory set up a VIP program where physicians administering the company's vaccines would receive points that could later be exchanged for VCRs, computers, and other expensive electronic equipment. The company withdrew the program under pressure from the Department of Health and Human Services, which cited a federal antikickback statute covering items reimbursed under Medicare and Medicaid, but only after many physicians had already participated.

Another program that continues today is that of the physicians' computer network. This is a nifty program. It is a consortium of 10 major drug companies that offers doctors a $35,000 office computer system, including hardware, software, printers, and maintenance, in exchange for access to all the medical records kept in the system. The doctors are asked to participate "in educational activities each month"; this requires a certain amount of reading of things that cross the screen. This computer network can track a physician's prescribing practices and patient information in intimate detail. Aside from the privacy issues, which I am sure have been resolved, it is a nifty bit of marketing for the drug companies because clearly it provides a handle on the doctor's prescribing patterns. The doctor gets a wonderful computer system. Is it a bribe? I don't know.

Perhaps the most infamous ploy is the frequent flyers program. I will just skip over that except to say that the program was banned in Massachusetts by a particularly aggressive attorney general who accused the company of fraud, leading to a $195,000 settlement and a lot of publicity. It continued in other states despite an investigation by the DHHS. The company does not like to talk about the program, and it does not reveal how many doctors received airline tickets, but a spokesman for American Airlines did tell Sidney Wolfe that "American Airlines said it was a very successful program from our standpoint."

An even less subtle marketing ploy cited by Wolfe is the outright offer of cash. Many drug companies provide large "grants for studies by doctors prescribing their drugs." Again, the word "studies" is put in quotation marks. The doctor uses the drug with 20 patients or so, reports the results in a brief questionnaire, and collects a check for $1,200 or more. Smaller sums are available for reading articles ($100 from Sandoz in exchange for reading a 3-page paper about the use of their versions of cyclosporin to treat psoriasis) and attending promotional dinners, $100 to $200 honoraria to pay for the doctor's time for listening to an evening talk about certain drugs.

In Britain, where physicians have been offered £500, or $1,000, to prescribe a new drug, such blandishments have not been entirely unsolicited. According to a report by the Royal College of Physicians, doctors have written to companies requesting money for foreign trips, even threatening to stop prescribing certain drugs unless their requests were granted. One group of physicians agreed to watch a promotional film on a new drug but stipulated that they had to be treated to dinner at a restaurant of their choice.

In one of the testimonies in the Senate hearings, a former public relations person at Abbott, David Jones, related some events that involved me in a peripheral way. In 1981, Merck was coming out with a new beta blocker called Blocadren®, and David Jones was at CIBA-GEIGY at the time. His company was marketing the beta blocker Lopressor®, which had the bulk of the market. CIBA-GEIGY was worried that Blocadren was going to take its market share away because Merck had sponsored a study that had to do with preventing heart attacks. It was a major, landmark study that received a great deal of publicity and was released in the *New England Journal of Medicine*.

I received a number of calls from a public relations company weeks in advance advising me to read my *New England Journal of Medicine* that week. I was also visited by CIBA-GEIGY, which wanted me to know that Lopressor, although it was not going to have a study released in the *New England Journal of Medicine*, was, in fact, already being used by doctors for this indication. I was informed that the research had been done and presented in a preliminary way and that I should write about that. In fact, I included that in my articles. When I went back to look at those articles, it was very clear to me that CIBA-GEIGY had a very good effect in making sure that I reported that Lopressor already existed and was the exact same kind of drug that was now being reported in the *New England Journal of Medicine*. One thing I did not realize was that, as David Jones reported in his testimony, I was not the only target for the marketing efforts. CIBA-GEIGY was giving out research grants to top cardiologists, sort of opinion makers in their regional areas, to conduct so-called clinical studies on Lopressor for the exact same purpose. Jones reported that the campaign had a tremendous effect on allowing Lopressor to keep its market share.

Now the big question is, does all of this promotion have any impact on physicians? The question is difficult to answer because prescription decisions are based on such a wide range of factors, including education, reading, study habits, patient request, reports from colleagues, idiosyncratic reports from personal experience, and a host of other influences of which doctors may not even be aware. Over the years, however, a number of researchers have attempted to determine the effects of advertising on doctors. One study of scientific versus commercial sources of influence on prescribing practices found that significant numbers of physicians favored the use of certain heavily promoted drugs. One example is the painkiller Darvon®. Despite scientific evidence and scientific literature that these drugs were risky and less effective than other available counterparts, the study concluded, physicians were strongly influenced by commercial nonscientific sources of drug information such as pharmaceutical sales representatives and manufacturers and advertisements, which can be misleading. Indeed, as one sales representative told a *New York Times* reporter, when there are eight drugs that are equally good, the doctor makes a choice based on nonscience; i.e., based on advertising and promotion.

There was research that assessed physicians' prescribing patterns before and after continuing medical education (CME) symposia. The research found that the sponsoring drug companies' products were prescribed more frequently over all after the symposium, despite the fact that CME courses are supposed to be unbiased objective sources of information on particular medical topics. Not surprisingly, the study also found evidence of significant bias in course content.

Finally, researchers have tried to correlate in some way the amount of impact and the effect of this impact with contacts between drug industry representatives and academic faculty and residents at seven major teaching hospitals in the Midwest. The researchers found that the house staff and faculty had an average of 1.5 conversations per month with a drug representative and that at least 25% had changed their prescribing practices as a direct result of such conversations.

The point is that there is something going on here. I think this kind of activity is heating up, and there also appears to be an interest on the part of the public–through Senate hearings, through other people, or through the press in particular–to begin publicizing this activity. I believe what the AMA decided is probably the beginning of a change in the trend; however, there is tremendous pressure in the industry to increase revenues during these competitive times. It is hard to tell exactly what is going on, but if you read the Pink Sheet, you will see several articles indicating congressional concerns about the various kinds of promotional efforts from the drug industry, what I would have to call a backlash by the politicians to some really troubling practices. For instance, Senator Pryor, who clearly is angry over what happened to his Medicaid bill, said in a speech that he was thinking of attacking the tax credits that pharmaceutical companies use for research. He questioned to what extent individual companies use the tax credits to write off what he called marketing research. Representative Stark said that he was going to look at the research and development credit that is being used three times more by the pharmaceutical industry than by manufacturing firms in general. He pointed out that he has sponsored legislation that would deny tax credits to drug firms that have excessive price inflation. Stark said that he was considering legislation to withhold any tax deductions for promotional materials not complying with FDA standards.

Finally, I just want to say that I do not begrudge the pharmaceutical industry's need to market its products. However, let me propose one abiding rule that seems to work across all other enterprises that I have covered as a journalist: avoid any conflict of interest and avoid even the appearance of a conflict. Be direct and truthful. If what you are doing is promotional, say so. An ad to the public, whether on television or in print, no matter if the message is also educational, is still an advertisement, and the public knows that. Tell the public why they are watching an ad. Tell them it is an advertisement for a drug. Finally, take some of the resources that are being used to promote drugs to doctors and the public and use them to tell your story better. I have been told that the Pharmaceutical Manufacturers Association has been trying aggressively to do this for years, but I have never seen it. Nobody in society begrudges high prices for high quality goods. All of us are willing to pay high prices when we know that what we are getting is worth the price. That's the message that should be remembered. The industry has plenty to be proud of, but it has also generated many questionable practices. I believe that if the industry can figure out a way to balance its actions, at least on its promotional side, all of us will benefit.

Pharmaceutical Advertising: Education versus Promotion

David G. Adams

It is a not-so-old adage that education has become big business in America. Today, a refinement may be in order. In the case of the American pharmaceutical industry, it appears that big business has become education.

Let us take the case of educational symposia for physicians. Senator Kennedy's Committee on Labor and Human Resources looked at the funding for educational symposia by a sampling of 16 drug companies in 1974 and 1988 (1). The committee found that in 1974, the companies spent approximately $6.5 million (in 1988 dollars) to sponsor approximately 7,500 educational symposia. For the year 1988, the committee reported an expenditure of $85 million in support of more than 34,000 educational symposia. We can surmise that even more is being spent today. It is a vast amount of money spent on a vast array of activities.

Not only has education become big business, but it has also become fun. It happens in some of the nicest places–Acapulco, Cancún, and, of course, that well-known center of higher education, Monte Carlo. As one of the brochures stated: "Monte Carlo is one of the most beautiful areas of the Côte d'Azur and an ideal venue for exchanging scientific ideas." This kind of education does not cost anything. The programs are free; lodging, meals, and transportation are provided. There are often impressive fringe benefits as well: all expenses paid for the physician's traveling companion; entertainment such as cruises, sailing, and golf; and cash honoraria. These are the scholarships of today's continuing medical education.

David G. Adams, J.D., is Associate Chief Counsel for Drugs for the United States Food and Drug Administration, 500 Fishers Lane, Room 689, Rockville, MD 20857.

The views expressed herein are those of the author and do not necessarily represent the position of the Food and Drug Administration.

53

Of course, education is not all fun and games, even in America and even in the case of health care products. I noticed in one recent brochure promoting an educational symposium that, packed in amidst the four days of fun and sun at a Florida resort, there were four hours of substantive presentations. I would assume that in these four hours the health care professionals were provided with information that they would find useful or interesting. One must assume that there is an opportunity for education here and, indeed, in most of the activities I have described. But, of course, there is also an opportunity for something else.

THE DIFFICULTY OF DISTINGUISHING EDUCATION FROM PROMOTION

Is it possible to distinguish education from promotion in a manner that would allow us to classify these activities as either one or the other? Can one totally separate promotional elements from educational elements in these activities? Good promotion should be educational to the extent that it provides useful information about the product offered for sale. Promotion, however, even if it is educational, must be considered a very special kind of education. The promoter is trying to get us to buy something. The educator is not trying to get us to buy something. Or is he? My dictionary defines education as the act or process of imparting or acquiring knowledge (2). The definition imposes no test of intellectual purity on the part of the educator.

Apparently, then, in the broadest sense of the words, promotion can involve education, and education can involve promotion. This means, of course, that the Food and Drug Administration (FDA) must become involved in regulating activities that are ostensibly educational. Where the educational activity involves promotion or is involved in promotion of drug products by those who market the products, the FDA has a regulatory interest because the FDA regulates the sale and promotion of drug products.

There are many kinds of ostensibly educational activities that have, to varying degrees, aroused the regulatory interest of the FDA. I will discuss three:

1. Educational activities sponsored by drug companies that are directed to health care professionals.
2. Educational activities sponsored by drug companies that are directed to consumers.
3. Educational activities by pharmacists.

Industry-Sponsored Education for Health Care Professionals

Physicians

Industry-sponsored educational activities for health care professionals are an area of major regulatory interest. These activities include, among others, programs and presentations such as lectures, workshops, and symposia. The agency has, over the years, become more concerned about these programs because of their scope and effectiveness as a promotional vehicle and because of the difficulty the agency has in regulating them. Because they are live events that are generally not reported to the agency by the sponsor, the agency seldom learns about them until the event is over. The agency has, however, asserted jurisdiction over these activities and is now in the process of developing a regulatory program to handle the illegal promotional aspects. I will return to this issue.

It has been somewhat easier for the agency to act on its regulatory interest in educational materials provided to health care professionals in written, printed, or graphic form. These are easier to come by. A good example is the supplement or special report in medical and scientific journals. In one recent case, the agency asserted jurisdiction over a special report on a study of a transdermal nitroglycerine infusion system. The agency's interest was aroused initially because the study was not blinded and because the study's suggestion of product efficacy was at odds with other, more reliable available data. The agency was also interested in the fact that the drug company that made the product had sponsored the study and had sponsored the special report supplement.

In another instance, the agency expressed concern over a report on a scientific meeting of the American College of Rheumatology. The report was provided to practitioners by a health care information service. Although many products were discussed at the meeting, the report focused on only one and focused particularly on the suggestion of a new indication for the product, an indication not approved by the FDA. As it happened, the information service that published the report had been paid by the drug company marketing the product to cover the meeting. The agency expressed a strong regulatory interest in both of these ostensibly educational activities.

Pharmacists

Although the educational activities I have discussed thus far have all been directed primarily to physicians, there have also been activities of interest to the FDA that have been directed to pharmacists. Although the industry-sponsored activities directed to pharmacists do not seem to involve all of the fun and games that generally accompany those directed to physicians (perhaps pharmacists are simply not as playful as physicians—I can only speculate), the industry has aroused the agency's regulatory interest in certain programs for pharmacists.

In one instance, the agency confronted a major pharmaceutical company with a transcript from a company-sponsored presentation provided to numerous local pharmacy association meetings. The agency found the presentation to be false and misleading in a way that favored the company's product over those of its competitors. The agency further objected to a letter-writing campaign by the company to pharmacists. These letters contained what the agency viewed as false and misleading claims concerning the product's absorption qualities. The agency threatened legal action against the company, and the activities were halted.

In another matter involving a different company, the agency objected to letters sent to pharmacists warning them that they faced potential liability if they substituted a generic drug for the company's brand-name product. The agency objected to the false and misleading nature of the company's claims, and the practice was halted.

Industry-Sponsored Activities
Directed to Consumers

Many drug companies desire not only to educate health care professionals, but also to educate consumers. And they want to educate consumers not only about over-the-counter (OTC) drugs, but also about prescription drugs. A prime example is the impressive effort by one major pharmaceutical firm to arrange the appearances of physicians on television talk shows to discuss the firm's new wrinkle cream. The firm's new wrinkle cream was approved by the FDA, of course, but not for wrinkles. The agency has expressed a regulatory interest in this matter.

Another firm, perhaps more attuned to consumer expectations on health care advice, sponsored the appearances on talk shows by a former baseball star to discuss the positive attributes of its nonsteroidal anti-inflammatory product. Although, in this instance, the product was approved for the suggested use, the agency found the presentation to be misleading and asserted a regulatory interest.

In another interesting case, a group of aspirin makers suggested the possibility of press conferences to present to the public new evidence on the beneficial effects of a daily aspirin regimen in preventing heart attacks in individuals who had not previously had a heart attack. Although this information was important, the agency was concerned that, for some individuals, the risk of having a heart attack might be less than the risk of other, harmful effects posed by the aspirin regimen. The agency impressed on the drug companies that this sort of education should come from physicians rather than from a press conference by an aspirin manufacturer.

Pharmacist Education of Consumers

Pharmacists, as well as drug companies, have potential liability under the act. Although the agency has taken little or no regulatory action involving pharmacist promotion or education in my recent memory, this is an area of regulatory interest, especially with regard to information on extra-label uses of drugs.

A few years ago, the agency was asked by a state health department to clarify whether a pharmacist can discuss with a physician or patient the use of an approved drug for an unapproved indication. The agency suggested that active, unsolicited promotion of an approved drug for an unapproved use would raise the prospect of a regulatory action by the agency.

THE FDA'S AUTHORITY TO REGULATE EDUCATION

How, one may ask, does the FDA purport to regulate pharmacists in providing information to consumers and physicians? How, for that matter, does the agency purport to regulate the industry-sponsored activities I mentioned? All of these activities may be viewed as educational in the broadest sense of that word. The answers to these questions are to be found in a few venerable provisions of the Federal Food, Drug, and Cosmetic Act (the act) (3). Passed by Congress in 1938, this legislation provides the FDA with the authority to regulate labeling and, per an amendment in 1962, advertisements for drug products. As interpreted by the FDA, these provisions provide means for reaching virtually all promotional activities for drug products.

In determining its regulatory approach to a promotional activity, the first question that the agency will consider is whether the activity can be regulated as labeling within the meaning of the act. This is because the agency's statutory authority over labeling is addressed with greater clarity and in greater detail than its authority over advertisements. In fact, with regard to OTC drugs, there is no express grant of statutory authority to regulate advertisements. The FDA reaches OTC drug ads through its legal authority to regulate OTC drug labeling.[1]

Jurisdiction over Labeling

One may reasonably ask how the FDA manages to regulate educational activities as labeling. None of the activities I have described here would appear to involve product labels. The answer to this question is to be found in the act's definition of labeling. This definition includes not only product labels, but also other written, printed, or graphic matter that accompanies a product. The scope of materials that are deemed to accompany a product has been broadly interpreted by the agency, as well as by the courts.[2] Materials can be deemed to accompany a product even though they are not actually provided with the product. If the materials are designed to supplement or explain the product, they are deemed to accompany it. They accompany the product not in the physical sense, but in the spiritual sense (4).

Consider, for example, professional labeling. This is information on OTC drugs that is provided only to health care professionals because it indicates uses that are inappropriate for self-diagnosis and self-medication by consumers. Formerly known as ethical advertising, these materials are now called professional labeling and are regulated under labeling provisions of the act, even though they do not physically accompany a product.

Jurisdiction over Advertisements

Of course, there are some activities that even the most creative agency lawyers cannot bring within the definition of labeling. Thus, we must consider the agency's authority to regulate advertisements. Interestingly, the act provides no definition for the term advertisement and contains only one statutory provision providing substantive requirements for advertisements.

What, then, is an advertisement? Congress did not define the term in the statute. The only hint in the statute as to the meaning of the term advertisement is the statement in the act that something that is labeling cannot be regulated as an advertisement.[3] The FDA has not defined the term in any regulation. Thus, I have no precise legal definition to offer. I do, however, have a good rule-of-thumb definition: in the view of the FDA, an advertisement is a promotional activity that cannot be regulated as labeling.

Under my rule-of-thumb definition, the key question is, when does the FDA regard an activity as promotional? Many people have said many things on this topic. I would describe the agency's regulatory approach as follows:

1. Those who sell drugs are responsible for the information they disseminate or cause to be disseminated with regard to their products.
2. This includes information disseminated to consumers as well as to intermediaries, such as health care professionals and the media. These intermediaries are persons who may be expected to pass the information on to consumers or, in the case of prescription drugs, to prescribe the products.
3. Those who sell drugs are responsible when they *sponsor* the dissemination of such information by other persons. This responsibility is based on their knowledge that they are sponsoring information on the products they sell. Sponsorship can include any substantial support, financial or otherwise, provided directly or indirectly by the seller of the drugs.

This assertion of jurisdiction may strike you as overbroad.

Could Congress have intended that the term advertisement include all these activities? Is the FDA simply taking advantage of Congress's failure to provide a precise definition in the statute for the term advertisement? As the FDA's attorney, I have argued that the agency is being true to the intent of Congress. The agency finds support for its interpretation in the legislative history of the prescription drug advertising provisions of the act.

In an early draft of the bill that was ultimately enacted as the 1938 act, Congress did provide a definition for the term advertisement. The term was defined to include "*all* representations of fact or opinion disseminated to the public in any manner or by any means other than labeling" (5). This sounds even broader than my proposed rule-of-thumb definition. Some in Congress apparently thought of the term advertisement as a rather far-reaching concept.

Constitutional Limitations

One might well ask at this juncture about the Constitution. Doesn't the First Amendment protect freedom of speech? Aren't there any limits on the FDA's ability to regulate the flow of information on drug products?

It is clear that in regulating labeling and advertisements, the government is regulating speech. It is, however, regulating a special kind of speech, known among lawyers as commercial speech. This form of speech, the Supreme Court has said on numerous occasions, is not entitled to the same protection as other types of speech.

Can the activities I have been discussing be deemed commercial speech? The answer appears to be "yes." The concept of commercial speech has not been limited to traditional advertising formats. The key factors that appear to determine whether speech can be regulated as commercial speech are (1) the commercial motivation behind the communication and (2) the reference to a specific product.

Once an activity is defined as commercial speech, as noted above, there is less constitutional protection. Commercial speech that is false or misleading enjoys no constitutional protection under the First Amendment. Even truthful commercial speech may be regulated if (1) the government has a substantial interest in the subject matter and (2) the regulatory approach reasonably fits the government's interest (6).

The government clearly has a substantial interest in regulating the sale and promotion of human drugs. The reasonableness of the agency's regulatory approach will, of course, depend on the facts. It is clear, however, that the FDA can regulate labeling and advertisements for drugs in a manner in which the government could never hope to regulate political speech.

Some may suggest that it is one thing to regulate information provided by *drug companies* as commercial speech, but it is quite another thing to suggest limits on constitutional protection for pharmacists when they provide information on drugs. Some may also question whether the agency can regulate those who give speeches under sponsorship of a drug company, especially if the speaker is an acknowledged expert who is expressing his or her sincerely held views.

Don't pharmacists and other experts have a constitutional right to express their views on drug products? The answer to this question must be qualified. Pharmacists, of course, sell drugs. Sometimes physicians also involve themselves directly in operations that sell drugs. There have been many examples, such as cancer clinics, acne clinics, and even hair growth clinics. When health care professionals are involved in both the sale and the promotion of specific products, the government cannot assume that there is no commercial motivation or aspect to their speech. This is not to denigrate the information provided by pharmacists and physicians or their professional integrity. It is simply not reasonable for government and courts to assume that because one is a professional, one has no commercial motivation.

What about experts who are sponsored by drug companies to express their personal opinions? They are not selling drugs. Or are they? Let us go back to the example I mentioned earlier involving the physician who is sponsored by a drug company to speak to pharmacists. Doesn't that physician have First Amendment rights? Again, the answer must be qualified.

Consider Dr. X, a well-known expert. Dr. X certainly has a right to express his views on drug products–views that a drug company selling those products might not have the same right to express. Does Dr. X have a constitutional right to have the drug company support or amplify his views, even though the company could not directly express such views? Could a drug company buy advertising time and, instead of hiring an actor to read a script, find an expert who likes the company's products and simply instruct the expert to go out and exercise his or her First Amendment rights by talking about the company's products?

In the view of the FDA, when a company chooses to amplify someone's views through the media, the company becomes responsible for the content. This position on the part of the agency may cause a company to forego support for the speaker's presentation. In this circumstance, the speaker may well believe that his or her First Amendment rights have been violated. This issue was actually litigated some years back in a case involving the late Carlton Fredericks, a well-known proponent of therapeutic uses of vitamins. The FDA had taken a legal action against the sponsor of Mr. Fredericks' radio program, in which he discussed therapeutic uses for the sponsor's products. Mr. Fredericks asserted that the government's legal action violated his First Amendment rights. The court did not agree. The company's refusal to sponsor Mr. Fredericks did not, in the view of the court, preclude Mr. Fredericks from presenting his views (7).

THE AGENCY'S DISTINCTION BETWEEN
PROMOTION AND EDUCATION

Is there, then, anything drug companies and pharmacists can say about the drug products they sell that will not be regulated as labeling or as an advertisement? There is. The FDA has acknowledged that drug companies and pharmacists have a role to play in educating health care professionals and consumers, a role that is not restricted by the labeling and advertising provisions of the act.

This is acknowledged, to some extent, in the FDA's regulations governing investigational uses for new drugs. The regulation first prohibits promotion–providing that a sponsor or investigator shall not make representations regarding the safety or effectiveness of the product under investigation if the statement is made in a promotional context (8). This provision is qualified, however, by a further statement that the regulation is not intended to restrict the full exchange of scientific information, including dissemination of scientific findings in scientific or lay media. This is an acknowledgement that researchers are good sources of information and that the agency does not want to inhibit unduly scientific exchange and will not necessarily regard such information as promotion. Pharmacists are not only good sources of information: giving information is a part of their professional responsibility.

Thus, there is an exception to the broad regulatory principles I have just been discussing, a recognition by the agency of an area of scientific exchange that will not be regulated as promotion. This is at the heart of what is generally referred to as the promotion/education distinction. It is a distinction that has been recognized in many of the contexts we have been discussing.

Lectures, Workshops, and Symposia

There are certain circumstances under which the FDA will not apply labeling and advertising provisions of the act to lectures, workshops, and symposia, even though the activities are supported by the drug companies whose products are discussed in the presentations. The agency will not object to sponsorship if it regards the activity as a bona fide scientific and educational activity and if the drug company has taken adequate steps to ensure (1) that the scientific/educational integrity of the program is maintained and (2) that the program does not become a vehicle for disseminating misleading or promotional information about a product marketed by the company.

The agency has suggested the following guidelines:

1. *It should be a true, scientific exchange.* The program should be presented by qualified experts. It should not be focused on or skewed in favor of a particular product of the sponsor. It should avoid extreme or fringe viewpoints and provide a medical context

for the views presented. It should not be directed to consumers. It should provide meaningful opportunities for exchange of scientific viewpoints.

2. *Care should be exercised in the discussion of unapproved uses.* Any such discussion should be in the context of a scientifically rigorous and objective discussion. The tone and emphasis should not be promotional. The information should be presented in the context of a larger body of data with adequate detail, and it should not promote the use of the product for the unapproved indication. The unapproved use should be described as such with proper emphasis on the limited nature of the current knowledge.

3. *Care should be exercised in making product comparisons.* The provider should attempt to ensure full and absolute objectivity and balance in terms of both content and emphasis of product comparisons. Such comparisons should be based on adequate and well-controlled studies. Suggestions of superiority should be supported by a rigorous and objective discussion.

4. *The format of the activity should avoid promotional elements.* In the view of the FDA, there should be no inducements provided to the attendees, other than meals and token gifts. There should be no undue focus on entertainment and leisure activities during the program.

5. *The sponsor's involvement should be disclosed.* The provider should disclose the sponsorship of the activity to the audience. Presenters should disclose significant financial or other relationships between themselves and the sponsor, including technical assistance provided by the sponsor for the presentation.

What about written reports on symposia or publications of studies themselves? The agency has allowed for the direct dissemination of scientific studies and other data and information by drug companies in certain limited circumstances; that is, where there is an unsolicited request for the information. If the detail man has suggested to the physician that he request such information from the company, the agency will regard the activity as promotional.

Company sponsorship of special reports and journal supplements discussing the company's products are more of a problem. The agency has, in the past, allowed many of these, but in examples I mentioned earlier, the agency found that the company was able to make the report or supplement into a promotional piece that was misleading or focused on unapproved uses. The agency will, I think, be focusing more regulatory attention on these matters in the foreseeable future.

Pharmacist Education of Consumers

The agency has tried to acknowledge a place for education within the practice of pharmacy similar to that acknowledged for drug companies. As noted above, the agency was asked by one of the state health departments to clarify whether a pharmacist can discuss with a physician or a patient use of an approved drug for an unapproved indication. The agency acknowledged that the line between regulated promotion and advising customers has always been a difficult one to draw. The agency has no regulations directed to this aspect of the practice of pharmacy, and the agency has traditionally handled the issue by not involving itself in pharmacists' advice to consumers. In its response to the state inquiry, however, the agency drew a distinction similar to that drawn with regard to the pharmaceutical industry. The agency noted its long-standing recognition of the scientific exchange and education and that it had no objection to pharmacists and drug companies providing information in response to *unsolicited requests* for information. I think the agency recognizes, of course, that in the context of the practice of pharmacy, where interaction between the pharmacist and consumers is informal, solicitation of information may be an imprecise concept.

As also noted above, the industry has sponsored efforts directing information on drugs to consumers. The agency has not acknowledged any role for industry in educating consumers outside of the labeling and advertising provisions of the act. Consumers are more vulnerable than health care professionals to promotion under the guise of education. The agency also has special concerns about industry efforts to promote prescription drugs to consumers. It is currently assessing its policy on allowing direct-to-consumer advertising and is planning to issue a policy statement in the near future. I think it is safe to assume that any information to consumers will continue to be regulated under the labeling and advertising provisions of the act.

WHERE TO FROM HERE?

It is possible to argue that any activity designed to provide information on drugs that is sponsored or carried out by a company or individual who sells the drugs should be regulated under the labeling and advertising provisions of the act, whether the activity is directed to consumers or to professionals. Indeed, some have argued that all of these activities, regardless of educational merit, *should be regulated* as promotion. They have also argued or acknowledged, however, that the current rules applicable to labeling and advertising must be changed to allow somewhat more flexibility for truly educational activities. That, of course, takes us back where we started.

The agency has acknowledged the important role played by drug companies and pharmacists in education and scientific exchange. If they are to continue to play a significant role, there must be a line drawn between activities held to the strict guidelines for promotion and activities held to less restrictive guidelines for education. This is the distinction that has traditionally been described as education versus promotion. This may or may not be the best way of describing the distinction. Lawyers can quibble over the description. The important issue is how the distinction is drawn.

For those involved in the sale of drugs, the standards by which their conduct is judged must be as clear as possible. This is important to individuals and companies who may be held civilly and criminally liable under the act. This is a matter of importance to the FDA as well, especially as the agency becomes increasingly committed to vigorous enforcement of the law with regard to drug promotion. In this regard, the agency is preparing, and expects to publish soon, a policy statement on industry-sponsored scientific and educational activities. This policy statement is intended to make the agency's regulatory approach to this area clearer to the industry. The agency is also considering the need for new regulations and, perhaps, new legislation.

Dr. Kessler's commitment to more vigorous enforcement in the area of drug advertising is clear and on the record. The promotional activities carried out in recent years under the guise of education are of special concern and, I predict, will be a high priority item for the foreseeable future. The issue we have described as promotion versus education is an issue whose time has come.

NOTES

[1]An OTC drug can be deemed to be misbranded under the act if it is not labeled for all of the intended uses of the product, including all uses for which the product is promoted in advertisements. See *Alberty Food Products v. United States*, 185 F.2d 321 (9th Cir. 1950). Thus, the FDA can reach claims made in advertising through its authority to regulate labeling.

[2] The term labeling is defined in Section 201(m) of the act, 21 U.S.C. 321(m), as "all labels and other written, printed, or graphic matter (1) upon any article or any of its containers or wrappers, or (2) accompanying such article." The act provides a separate, narrower definition for the term label: "a display of written, printed, or graphic matter upon the immediate container of any article . . . ," Section 201(k), 21 U.S.C. 321(k).

[3] The agency's authority over advertisements, set forth in Section 502(n) of the act, 21 U.S.C. 321(n) (the only provision of the act in which the term advertisement is used), is expressly limited to materials and activities that do not fall within the act's definition of labeling.

REFERENCES

1. Science Policy Research Division. Congressional Research Service. Library of Congress. Memorandum to Senator Edward Kennedy. 9 December 1990.

2. Random House college dictionary. rev. ed. New York: Random House, 1975.

3. The act is codified at 21 U.S.C. §§ 301-92.

4. *Kordel v. United States*, 335 U.S. 345 (1948).

5. S. 5, 74th Congress, 1st Session (1935).

6. *Board of Trustees of SUNY v. Fox*, 109 S.Ct. 3028 (1989).

7. *United States v. Articles of Drug . . . Century Food Co.*, 1938-1964 FDLI Judicial Record 1796 (S.D. Ill. 1963).

8. 21 CFR 312.7(a).

Some Comments
on Direct-to-Consumer Advertising

Robert A. Ingram

Let me share some thoughts on pharmaceutical promotion–and specifically offer some comments on direct-to-consumer advertising–from Glaxo's perspective.

I am sure many people are familiar with the comment by Sir William Osler, the Canadian physician: "Care for the patient is best served by care for the patient." Of course he meant that health care is best delivered when the physician and pharmacist are truly concerned about their patient's well-being. I submit that Osler's thought can be extended to my company.

Sure, our industry cares about the bottom line. What business or individual does not? But if you take a hard, honest look beyond the bottom line, I think almost everyone in the industry–indeed, almost everyone in any health-related profession–chose his or her career at least in part because it is one that makes a difference to people. And if we in industry take another hard look, I think we can see clearly the value of what we do. We can see the true value of medicines to society and to individual patients, a topic I will return to later. That is part of what makes our business so rewarding. As Mike Waldholz said, it is also a story we have kept to ourselves far too long.

I know our critics will claim that this is just public posturing by another greedy industry spokesman. My only response to that is: they're wrong. As corny as it may sound, I know in my heart that we're in an important, valuable, even noble business. And I hope anyone considering our motives will at least keep an open mind about what we are attempting to accomplish. Of course, the more you listen to the public pronouncements of the so-called industry watchdogs, the more you appreciate the

Robert A. Ingram is Group Vice President at Glaxo Inc., Five Moore Drive, Box #13398, Research Triangle Park, NC 27709.

67

wisdom of the old adage–the one that says knowledge without understanding is like heat without light. And I can attest that the temperature in our industry is warming considerably. But when we cast light on the situation, I think it is clear that promotion by *responsible* pharmaceutical companies has always put the patient first. As I said before, our actions in this area are driven by both social and business needs. In our industry, a business that does not put the patient first will not remain in business for long.

So let's extend that thought for a moment. If we believe, with Osler, that the best way to care for the patient is to care for the patient, and if we believe that care is best delivered by a well-informed physician and a well-informed pharmacist to a well-informed patient, then we must also believe that we must do nothing to interfere with the doctor-pharmacist relationship. This, then, is one of the basic tenets guiding our promotion. We firmly believe that the physician is the best judge of a course of treatment for a patient and that each physician and patient should have access to every means of treatment available.

The first step in selecting a treatment, obviously, is knowing about it, understanding its benefits and drawbacks–and *THAT* is the function of promotion. I know we have already discussed education versus promotion. Fully realizing that there are differing opinions in this room, I suggest that if the promotion is done responsibly–through truth well told–the concepts are one and the same.

But wait, our critics would say, you cannot sell and educate at the same time. I disagree. And I offer as proof our now-concluded direct-to-consumer campaign on peptic ulcer disease to which Mike Waldholz has referred. Mike may not have pointed out that it began after a survey of antacid users revealed that although many were overmedicating, many were not planning a visit to the doctor. As you heard, the ads were not product-specific; they didn't mention Zantac®, our ulcer medicine, but instead focused on disease awareness. They pointed out that chronic use of antacids may be dangerous, they alerted consumers that doctors can prescribe treatment programs to cope with chronic stomach pain, and they encouraged sufferers to seek medical treatment.

Did it educate? As Mike mentioned, the ads in the 2 1/2-year campaign were seen by 12 million people and generated over 580,000 visits to physicians. Did it sell? Yes, a portion of those visits did result in prescriptions for Zantac, although, again, the ads did not mention Zantac by name, and they were prescriptions that the physicians deemed appropriate and that answered patients' needs. The point is that educating, caring for patients, advertising, and, yes, selling are not mutually exclusive activities.

And I would even go a step further to say these are activities that are increasingly valuable to our society. For example, how many of those 580,000 people would have continued their self-medication, risking the expense and trauma of surgery? How many days of work would have been missed? How much productivity lost? How much would this have added to the nation's total health care costs?

In fact, the value of responsible promotion has been recognized by no less an authority than Food and Drug Administration (FDA) Commissioner Kessler, who, before he accepted the FDA post, coauthored an article that appeared in the *Journal of the American Medical Association*. Dr. Kessler wrote: "Those who question promotional activities need to recognize that they have value, are here to stay, and will continue to be a major source of information about prescription drugs." In fairness to Dr. Kessler, he went on to say, "But those who argue for further expansion of these activities, especially of direct-to-consumer advertising, must exercise caution." I would add that it is a matter of whether we want to regulate ourselves or be regulated.

Will the industry benefit? Probably. Will the patient benefit? Absolutely. And yes, there are risks involved. But risks are at the very heart of the research-based pharmaceutical industry. Everyone who has been a part of research and development (R&D) budget deliberations knows that. And if experience has taught us anything in this industry, it is that standing still is tantamount to moving backward.

I, for one, have always relied on experience. It lets me recognize a mistake every time I make it. In this case, however, experience tells me that it would be a mistake not to investigate more fully the benefits of direct-to-consumer advertising. At the same time, we must be aware of the potential for mistakes *UNLESS*-and this is an important qualifier-unless the ads are well thought out and conceived with the purpose of getting patients together with the physicians equipped to serve them. In Glaxo's view, this principle must be one that guides any direct-to-consumer advertising our industry undertakes. Another is that the information in the ad must be truthful. As David Adams said, "Companies must be responsible for *all* the information we disseminate."

Many, no doubt, read the comments of Dr. Sidney Wolfe of the Public Citizen Health Research Group as reported in the *New York Times*. Speaking about consumer ads sponsored by pharmaceutical companies, he said: "These ads are raw naked appeals to people's pain. I want people to challenge their doctors based on good information, but these ads are misinformation or even false information."

Well, that is absurd. First of all, Glaxo simply would not do that. But putting ethical considerations aside, I suggest that advertising of any sort, and health care advertising particularly, contains a built-in brake against falsehood. If a product does not do what it says it will, there is no chance for a repeat sale. In pharmaceutical advertising, we have another safeguard: a physician must think it necessary before a consumer can buy the product. But in any case, one falsehood brings an entire promotional plan to a screeching halt. It's sort of like the tourist who asked the Grand Canyon guide if people often fell over the cliff. "No," the guide answered, "once is usually enough." If we depart from the truth in any way, I am sure we will find the precipice steep and the landing extremely unpleasant.

So the ads must be truthful, and that is really the easy part. But they also must be useful, and that is a little harder to achieve. How much information should they contain? How should information on benefits and side effects be presented? How technical should the language be?

I have no proof, but my personal feeling is that we underestimate the sophistication of the consumer. Patients today are becoming vocal advocates for quality, cost-effective care. These days, when the media blanket us with medical news and when the *Physicians' Desk Reference* is a part of many home libraries, consumers are starving for medical information. If it affects their health, I believe they agree with Samuel Johnson that "all knowledge is valuable; there is nothing so inconsiderable that I would rather not know it." And I suggest to those who would withhold health care information because they think that patients are incapable of understanding it or that they will misuse it that such an attitude deprives the patient of the dignity he deserves. I further submit that it demeans the quality of care.

I believe it is clear that consumers see value in health care information from any source, including ads by prescription pharmaceutical companies. A 1989 study by Scott-Levin Associates suggested that the ads fill a genuine need. In that study, more than 70% of consumers said they believed that direct-to-consumer ads are an important and valuable educational tool and that they are a source of reliable health care information. The report also said that when patients ask about a specific drug, doctors agree the requests are usually appropriate. Over 70% of the physicians in the survey said that patients asking about a drug actually did suffer from a condition the drug was designed to treat. Perhaps more significantly, 17% of the physicians had diagnosed a disease as a result of a patient coming in and describing symptoms seen in an ad. I think you would have a hard time convincing those patients that the ads were not useful. Far from interfering in the physician-patient relationship, the ads appear to facilitate it *IF*–and this is another important qualifier–the planners of the campaign have done their homework and their legwork.

Before any ad is launched, the company must do a thorough job of its professional communications. Through journal ads, sales representative visits, medical meetings, and other means, we must first answer any questions physicians and pharmacists may have about our medicine. All of our messages must be scrupulously prepared and be created in consultation with federal regulators. We at Glaxo have benefited from the counsel of Ken Feather and David Banks. Then we must begin a dialogue with physicians and pharmacists about any about-to-be-launched campaign. We would certainly be helping no one–least of all ourselves–if we created a situation in which patients began asking questions that their physicians and pharmacists could not answer.

The way we see it, if the ads are prepared and presented responsibly, they enhance the interaction among physicians, pharmacists, and patients. Apparently, more and more individual physicians are beginning to agree, despite the fact that most medical organizations take the opposing view. For example, in the Scott-Levin study, most said non-product-specific ads that direct a consumer to contact a doctor (like Glaxo's peptic ulcer disease awareness campaign, which I mentioned earlier) were appropriate. On the other side of the coin, only a few said it was appropriate to mention medicines by name. This is more evidence, I submit, of the huge, flashing caution light towering before this issue.

Nevertheless, the numbers indicate an apparently growing acceptance of direct-to-consumer advertising by both patients and physicians. So why the controversy? Why are some observers so sure that the ads are harbingers of calamity, while others equate their significance with the discovery of fire?

I do not have the answers. And from time to time I think it is a shame that the only people who know all the answers are so busy driving taxicabs, cutting hair, and writing newspaper editorials. In any case, I suspect it is at least partly because we are simply breaking new ground.

The advertising we know and are comfortable with–that is, the advertising directed to physicians and pharmacists and approved by regulators–may not be appropriate for a lay audience. Everyone's a little nervous, including industry, about sending the right message to consumers. It will require careful thought and give and take on the part of all of us to work out this issue. But I have no doubt that we will work it out to the benefit of the patient and to the benefit of us all. And I am sure that those messages will be responsible and appropriate. I am sure they will not repeat the images and the themes of the ads for the nostrums of the nineteenth and early twentieth centuries, images that, unfortunately, haunt us today.

Bill Reynolds has discussed the history of medical advertising, so I am sure you know what I am referring to. Advertising copywriters created ads like the one first published in 1888 for Dr. Owen's Body Battery, which created an electric current that the ad copy said "can be applied to any part of the body or limbs by the whole family. Cures general, nervous and chronic diseases. Guaranteed for one year." The real shock, of course, was felt in your wallet. We have come a long way since the Body Battery. And while we should be mindful of the unfortunate advertising legacy of yesterday's snake-oil salesmen, we cannot allow ourselves to be paralyzed by it. Instead, we should be bold enough to learn from the past and build on our successes.

Today we do not need to discover diseases for our medicines to treat. Unfortunately, the world has too many legitimate ones for us to treat. These diseases include hypertension, arthritis, and ulcer disease, each less of a threat today because of our industry's efforts. Indeed, it is the pharmaceutical industry that is regularly providing true breakthroughs to meet these and other genuine unmet patient needs. This does not happen as often as we would like, perhaps, but our record remains admirable. And not insignificantly, this is one of the ways in which our products have demonstrated their value.

If you suffered from cardiac disease, would you rather be treated with a tablet or with $30,000 bypass surgery? If you suffered from ulcers, would you prefer a tablet or the surgeon's blade? If you were being treated with chemotherapy for cancer, would you rather experience the violent retching that may follow or take a medicine that allows you to go back to work and have a chili dog for lunch?

These breakthroughs, by the way, have not contributed to burgeoning health care costs as significantly as recent headlines would have you believe. That may sound surprising, but it is nonetheless true if you look at how the health care dollar is actually spent. In 1987, for example, 67¢ of every dollar was spent on hospital care and physicians' services. Only 5¢ went to prescription drugs. From 1965 to 1989, the percentage of the United States' GNP devoted to *health care* jumped from 6% to about 11%. But percentage of GNP to *prescription drugs* remained constant at less than 1%. So despite what you might hear in a bar outside Riverfront or on the floor of the Senate, these are a few reasons why modern pharmaceuticals remain such a good value. They truly are the best and most cost-effective value in health care.

Enough of my soapbox. But this does have a direct bearing on pharmaceutical promotion and advertising. Because in today's environment, it is not enough for the industry to provide only the breakthrough medicines I just mentioned. We must also provide the information people need to take advantage of those medicines.

In this area, industry and pharmacy are uniquely positioned to help each other. While physicians and the industry must share the burden of providing the information that today's consumers demand, it is the pharmacist who is on the front lines. It is the pharmacist who is in the best position to explain to the patient how a medicine works, how to take it, and what to expect in terms of effects and side effects. And to the often-asked question–what makes this tiny bottle of medicine worth $65?–the pharmacist is in the ideal position to explain that if it is taken correctly, if it cures an illness or avoids a more serious condition later on, it is the best investment in health a patient could hope to make. It is up to the pharmacist to explain that the most expensive prescription is the one taken inappropriately or not at all. I suggest that such explanations are not only in the patient's best interests, but also in the pharmacist's best interests, too.

Beyond that, however, I think pharmacists would welcome more involvement with patients because undeniably that is where the action is, especially in these days of heightened consumer activism. That is where pharmacists can use their considerable skills in the science of pharmacology and the art of human relations.

The result is a more knowledgeable consumer. And a knowledgeable consumer treated by a knowledgeable physician and counseled by a dedicated pharmacist will lead to better doctor-pharmacist-patient interactions and better patient compliance: in short, better care. And importantly, that will help maintain an environment in which industry can continue investments in R&D–investments that will lead to the next generation of breakthroughs for ourselves and our children. This will, of course, lead to even better care in the future.

Now that I have spent so much time describing the possible controversial future of pharmaceutical promotion, let me leave you with another thought. Is a controversy inevitable? Doesn't everyone agree that a responsibly informed patient is a better patient? How far apart are the players in this issue anyway?

I am reminded of a story told by an advertising executive about a team of neurosurgeons standing around an operating table, several hours into an incredibly delicate brain surgery. The chief surgeon is sweating profusely in his blood-spattered gown. He sighs wearily and asks for his brow to be wiped. He steps away for a moment's rest, and finally a colleague grabs him by the shoulders and shouts, "Get hold of yourself, man! It's not like we're doing advertising." While we are not talking about brain surgery, we are dealing with an area of health care that may have consequences that are just as great. I am confident that all of us–physicians, pharmacists, legislators, regulators, and industry–will proceed in a manner that best serves the patient.

Pharmaceutical promotion has had an interesting past; I am sure it will have an interesting future. But as Emerson said, "What lies before us and what lies behind us are small matters compared to what lies within us." That is why I am certain that whatever the form of future promotion, the patient will be the winner. I am certain that what lies within every member of the health professions is a desire for quality patient care. That, after all, is why we are here.

New Directions
in Pharmaceutical Advertising

John Vandewalle

Advertising in the pharmaceutical industry goes back many eons, and for a long while, it has been somewhat stereotyped, with most of the effort being directed to the print media. With the new technological revolution today, there is an advertising revolution under way in the pharmaceutical marketplace. In this article, the tactical approaches in the form of new technologies will be addressed, but the emphasis will be on the strategic approach as the new direction in pharmaceutical advertising.

PHARMACEUTICAL ADVERTISING: A DEFINITION

Advertising is defined as "making generally or publicly known" or "describing publicly with the view to increasing sales." Both public relations and print advertising fall under this umbrella, and although there are differences in execution and perception, both of these approaches share common goals.

All advertising assists in meeting corporate goals and appears in the media. Direct advertising creates brand recognition by delivering key messages with control and predictable frequency. It has limitations, including the high cost of advertising space, the inflexibility of the medium once in print, and limited credibility associated with direct advertising. Public relations, on the other hand, while lacking the control and predictability of direct advertising, can often deliver a message with full credibility. It is acknowledged as "independent, unsponsored material" that reflects the view of freelance reporting.

John Vandewalle, M.D., is Director of Global Commercial Development at Marion Merrell Dow Inc., in Kansas City, MO 64114.

75

There are a number of elements of a pharmaceutical product that contribute to its advertising profile. These are, among others:

- The Name–how it sounds and how easily the name can be recalled and written.
- The Image–what differentiating features of the product are remembered by way of promotional message, including efficacy and safety?
- The Price–is this an identifying feature that overwhelms the image?
- The Presentation–how it looks, how it feels, and what comes with it.
- The Acceptance–how is it accepted by the customer, be it the prescriber or the end-user parties involved in the chain of events required to get the product to its final destination?
- The Support–who and what are the backers of the product?

While these elements are nothing new to us, too often they are allowed to evolve independently, in the absence of a holistic vision for the final product image. The result is often a collage or chimera rather than a well-architectured mosaic. Too often the puzzle is patched together with disjointed pieces, in contrast to being the intended outcome of a well-integrated plan.

FORCES OF CHANGE IN PHARMACEUTICAL ADVERTISING

In the wake of the technological revolution, there are other environmental issues that are forcing a revolution in the approach to pharmaceutical advertising. These issues include the dissolution of political boundaries, the formation of economic coalitions, the enlargement of the management domain, the creation of the universal audience, and the realization that illness and knowledge have no boundaries.

The dissolution of political boundaries, such as that occurring in the European community, is fostering more interaction and is leading to the formation of consortiums of regulatory bodies and health authorities. A central regulatory body in Europe is no longer just a subject of future speculation. The inclusion of foreign data in an NDA in the U.S. is becoming more accepted. Pharmacovigilance now extends beyond the confines of single countries. Global distribution of pharmaceutical products and their intermediates is increasing. Legal requirements for scientific data protection and patent respect are becoming more universal, as are the rights of patients. The litigious fever is escalating and crossing national boundaries. Sponsors are being held responsible for the products they export.

With the formation of economic coalitions, pricing of products around the world is becoming more transparent. Cost-containment programs are well entrenched and are here to stay. Gone are the times of free pricing opportunities for pharmaceutical products. Pricing itself has become a new science that is expanding rapidly during a time when pharmacoeconomic justification is considered a priority. Today a justification for a particular price tag on a product is paramount to the acceptance of products into formularies, to acceptance by prescribers, and, to an increasing degree, to acceptance by the patients who are required to pay for a greater portion of their therapy.

In this era of supersonic transportation, the management domain has extended well beyond the office or the territory in a country and is no longer constrained by national mores. The purview of the providers, prescribers, and recipients is only limited by the constraints of money, time, or motivation. Multinational organizations bring together cross-cultural management, and international congresses serve as coliseums for the world. International travel has allowed for cross-cultural interaction and has led to the reduction of territorial imperatives, to increased awareness of common denominators, and to a new drive toward harmonization.

As much as international travel has contributed to the revolution, advances in communication technologies have contributed even more. Radio, for example, in the forms of Voice of America, British Broadcasting Corporation, and Physicians Radio Networks has become a major medium for reaching audiences interested in health care. Television has now become the global box office and yields formidable power through its coverage, appeal, diversity, and flexibility. Television stations such as CNN and Eurochannel are representative of more than just national opinion. In the appeal to wider audiences, television has developed common themes and messages that generate tremendous hype and momentum. Pharmaceutical marketers have taken advantage of the medium to deliver their messages to the homes of receptive prescribers and patients. In some cases, customized television is appealing to the medical fraternity. An example of this is Lifetime Medical Television in the U.S. Direct-to-consumer advertising, which generally promotes awareness of a disease, induces visits to individual doctors or clinics and is a relatively new avenue that is being adopted with success.

Today the videotape is serving as a mainstream educational portal for the prescriber, and very often for the lay public, offering information on patient management, specific drugs and treatment, and highlights of personal interviews and congresses. Videotape is almost the ideal promotional format because it can be customized for primary and secondary target audiences. It has greater impact in that it appeals to two faculties, sight and sound, and can simplify complex messages or embellish simple messages.

The print medium, which has been the mainstay of advertising and academic presentations for decades, is now also moving across nations into the far corners of the earth. The *New England Journal of Medicine* (*NEJM*), the *British Medical Journal* (*BMJ*), *Lancet*, and the *Journal of the American Medical Association* (*JAMA*) are just a few examples of what might be called international medical journals. As far as the lay press is concerned, tabloids such as the *Wall Street Journal, Financial Times, International Herald Tribune*, and *Time* have a broad reach. These are vehicles in which advertising can be deployed for far-reaching impact.

Telecommunications, including systems such as telefaxing, teleconferencing, and computer data transmission via modem, are bringing information to the doorsteps of newly accessible audiences.

But what is the end result of all of this? Who is at the end of the communication chain or at the center of the communication web? The patient is the final recipient of this information, either directly or indirectly, when this information is transformed into a health service of some nature.

MANAGING THE REVOLUTION IN PHARMACEUTICAL ADVERTISING: A CORE COMMERCIALIZATION PROGRAM

Leaders in the pharmaceutical industry are aware of the new technologies and other trends influencing globalization and of the challenges and opportunities they are facing. To optimize results in globalization, corporations must concentrate on issues beyond geography. At Marion Merrell Dow (MMD), a core commercialization program has been implemented to facilitate global teamwork and to create and implement global plans. A core program is a flexible umbrella management system with two major components: (1) the core team or core group and (2) the core plan (Figure 1).

The Global Commercial Development Department at MMD is responsible for managing the core team, which consists of members from cross functional areas including research, development, manufacturing, commu-

FIGURE 1.

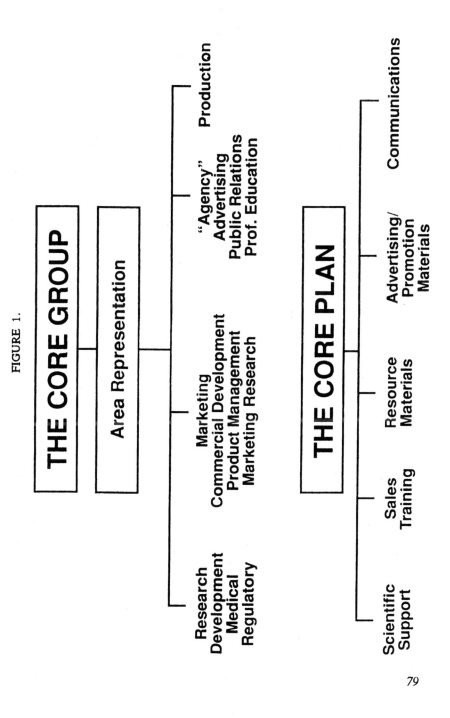

THE CORE GROUP

Area Representation

Research
Development
Medical
Regulatory

Marketing
Commercial Development
Product Management
Marketing Research

"Agency"
Advertising
Public Relations
Prof. Education

Production

THE CORE PLAN

Scientific
Support

Sales
Training

Resource
Materials

Advertising/
Promotion
Materials

Communications

nications, regulatory, and legal. Each global geographic area is represented by associates on the core team. The core team is responsible for developing a core plan that includes a clinical operating plan, adapts a global regulatory strategy, seeks a global trademark, fosters a global pricing strategy, provides global positioning, rolls out a global forecast, and reflects the plans for global communications. The plan is made up of the documentation that supports the activities of the group. This is used as the road map for the corporation and the individual countries for developing and commercializing the product.

The program is not cast in iron and handed down to the implementers through the tiers of the organization. It is a flexible management plan that has input and buy-in from those in the corporation who are identified as key strategic experts as well as key implementation experts. Full participation and buy-in is critical to the successful global effort.

To begin the process, compounds are funneled from research and licensing opportunities to a New Business Committee (Figure 2). Already, at this early stage, Global Commercial Development is involved in providing information with regard to commercial opportunities and compound naming. This allows for compound characterization in a field of commercial interest. If the compound has a clear pathway through Phase II, the New Business Committee reviews the compound and decides on approving the compound for clinical development. Once approval is given, the global strategy is compiled, and the product is developed and commercialized according to that strategy. The core team is responsible for nurturing the product to the market globally.

To illustrate the process, a case study is presented below. It presents a product with the generic name of vigabatrin and the trade name of Sabril®.

SABRIL: A CASE STUDY

The concept of vigabatrin arose from the knowledge of Marion Merrell Dow scientists that seizures result from inhibition of the synthesis of gamma aminobutyric acid (GABA), an inhibitory neurotransmitter, as well as from administration of GABA receptor antagonists. Vigabatrin was synthesized as a rational approach to manipulate the GABA system. It is a specific irreversible inhibitor of GABA transaminase, which results in enhanced levels of GABA in the synaptic cleft. The product was named Sabril, and this trademark was registered in all but three countries where the drug is intended to be marketed, among them are the U.S., France, Italy, the U.K., Germany, and Japan. While the product has yet to be introduced in the U.S., the U.S. is part of the core package.

FIGURE 2.

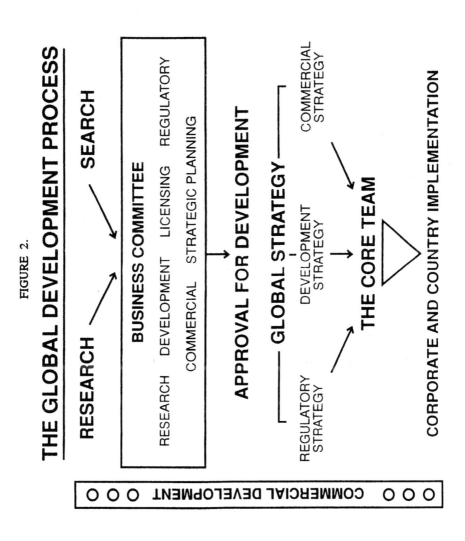

THE GLOBAL DEVELOPMENT PROCESS

During the first stages of the development of the core package, regulatory and clinical development strategies were devised and expedited. Then, with respect to commercial development, the standard market research was instituted simultaneously in the major countries around the world. The market was assessed in terms of competition and therapeutic areas. This allowed Marion Merrell Dow to get a good fix on the total market and to dissect this market into the various subsectors (Figure 3). The market research was then rerun. The second time, a product concept was tested in the same countries, and a universal product positioning was developed.

With the product positioning in place and serving as the foundation stone for the marketing strategy, the marketing concepts could be developed. Proposals were developed giving special consideration to the fact that more than 15 years had transpired since the availability of a new antiepilepsy drug, the mechanism of action of the older drugs remains uncertain, and there are patients who are not adequately controlled on traditional therapy. Four themes were identified in the positioning, and these were used as the guidelines for the development of the global marketing concepts, which were then researched in the same major countries (Figure 4).

One concept, "A new era of seizure control starts here . . . with the rationally designed antiepileptic Sabril," became the clear choice (Figure 5). It was selected because doctors felt that it had a strong positive impact and was original and relevant to the product and to the field of therapy. Doctors felt that the pin shown in the advertisement added to the intended message of efficacy by illustrating the "start of therapy and point of control." This marketing concept then served as the template for the development of all of the other materials. Other materials included a prelaunch advertisement, a product monograph, an advertisement to the family physician, and a host of other materials, as well as a corporate advertisement where the molecule is depicted chemically and the pin is subtly introduced.

Final steps in the process include promotional material testing; market acceptance studies, including pricing studies; and a reevaluation of the quantitative market data.

CONCLUSION

In summary, the global development strategy is achievable if the approach is through the team, the focus is on the product, the national boundaries are dissolved, and the national interests are respected. The

FIGURE 3.

ANTI-EPILEPTIC MARKET – GLOBAL

Leading Compounds
(Sales – 000 $)
Total Global Market: $641 MM (MAT 3Q89)

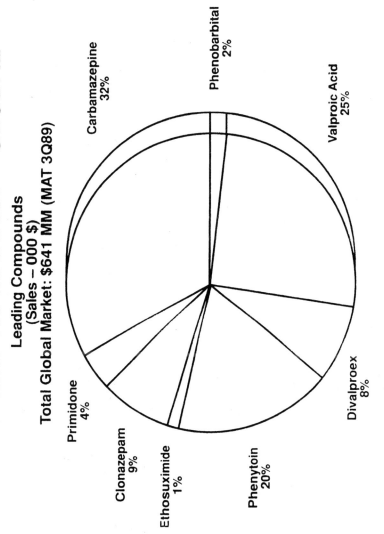

FIGURE 4.

VIGABATRIN
SABRIL

POSITIONING

PRODUCT POSITIONING STATEMENT

FOUR THEMES WERE IDENTIFIED
FOR FURTHER ELABORATION:

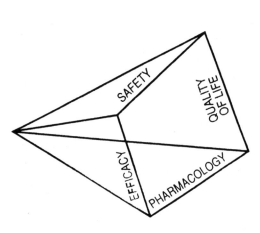

FIGURE 5.

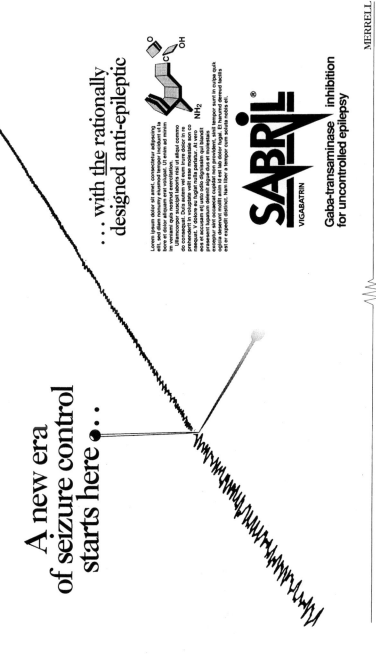

85

philosophy must be clearly understood there, and the commitment must be etched in stone. The license for operation must be vested in a coordinating body that is charged with the delivery of a global uniform message.

At the outset, every obstacle will appear in the path of success, and there will be more advocates of doom than triumph. But once successful, the process will engender commitment to the approach. Dignity, equity, respectability, and a global franchise will then have been acquired for a product as well as for the corporation supporting it.

Trends in Health Care Consumer Communications

Wayne L. Pines

A discussion of trends in consumer health care communications carries with it the risk of being instantly out of date. This is a field that is moving so quickly, in which change is so dynamic, that anything said one month may well be more historical than current in a very short period of time. The reason for this is that our health care system itself is undergoing continued significant change, both technologically as well as financially; consumers' interest in their own health continues to intensify, especially as the population ages; the expectations of the public of advances in health care continue to be high; the technology by which messages can be delivered to consumers continues to become more sophisticated; and the competition among pharmaceutical and other health care companies is such that every advantage, including communications advantages, will be sought.

I am going to focus on the provision to consumers of information about prescription drugs, especially on the role that pharmaceutical companies have played in consumer communications and the prospects for expanded efforts.

Some initial historical perspective may be appropriate. It was not too long ago that consumer interest in health care generally, and prescription drugs specifically, was far less intense than it is today. When I was growing up, my family had a doctor-Dr. Friedman-who took care of our medical needs. When we were sick, Dr. Friedman came to our home and treated us with medicines that he pulled out of a black bag. Except for drugs like penicillin, no one really knew the names of the drugs we were receiving or what side effects we might encounter. If I wanted to know anything about a drug, I would hesitate to ask Dr. Friedman, figuring

Wayne L. Pines is Executive Vice President of Burson-Marsteller, 1850 "M" Street, NW, Washington, DC 20036.

that his time was too precious and that I probably would not understand. My local pharmacist was friendlier and more helpful, but the world of prescription drugs was still unexplored territory for me and just about everyone else without a health care background.

Further, when Dr. Friedman treated us, my parents paid the bill directly to him, and when we needed a prescription, we paid the pharmacist directly. Medical care was simpler and less expensive in those days. It also was less effective. People died earlier, and when people did live with illness, the quality of their lives, especially the elderly, was poorer.

Since those days, there has been a revolution in the capability of our health care system to maintain our health and quality of life. There also has been a revolution in how health care is delivered and in the information desired by and available to consumers about prescription drugs, other therapies, and diagnostic procedures.

Doctors do not make house calls anymore because it is not economical and because they have equipment in their offices that helps them diagnose diseases more efficiently and accurately. Indeed, many consumers, especially in our mobile society where one out of five people moves each year, do not even have family physicians like Dr. Friedman. Instead, they rely on a series of specialists or coordinate their health care themselves.

There are new drugs introduced virtually every year to treat diseases that were incurable a generation ago. From a personal health standpoint, consumers have a greater interest in directing their own health care. There are many signs of this: physical fitness is now big business, the *Physicians' Desk Reference* (*PDR*) is a best-seller, the bookstores are filled with other health books, and many people can now discuss intelligently with their physicians surgical procedures or treatment choices. There is also a willingness on the part of the government and the medical community to permit more drugs to move from prescription to over-the-counter (OTC) status, placing more responsibility and power in the hands of consumers.

Financing of health care has also changed. Payment methods have undergone a radical change. More and more people are enrolling in health maintenance organizations (HMOs). Many others have their bills paid by the government under Medicare or Medicaid. Those who work are usually covered by complicated insurance plans, and unfortunately, a significant number of people, by virtue of their lack of insurance coverage, are denied access to a health care system that is at once the world's most sophisticated and most expensive. Finally, another new factor in medicine relates to a defensive approach to medical practice due to product liability concerns. This approach can translate into unnecessary testing and increased costs.

The reason I begin with this historical perspective is that it is important to understand the larger context in which information about prescription drugs has been available to consumers. The changes that have occurred in health care consumer communications are a natural fallout of the changes that have occurred in the quality of our health care, the consumer's unprecedented interest in personal health, and the consumer's access to the health care system.

I focus now on health care communications. There are many milestones that can be cited to illustrate and underscore the changes that have taken place in this area over the past two or three decades. I would like to mention just one because it was one I observed and, in fact, covered as a reporter. That was the decision in the early 1970s by the Food and Drug Administration (FDA) to require a patient package insert (PPI) for oral contraceptives. That PPI truly was a historical breakthrough.

In the early 1970s, a Wisconsin senator, Gaylord Nelson, held frequent hearings involving medical issues, and one of his favorite topics was oral contraceptives (OCs). Senator Nelson was assured of getting major headlines from his hearings because there was an insatiable public thirst for more information about drugs like OCs, and there were few sources then available.

The FDA made a courageous decision at the time in the context of the Nelson batterings. It decided that since OCs were elective drugs–drugs not used to treat a traditional disease, but taken by healthy people–there was a legitimate role for the patient in deciding whether to take the drug. That might sound elementary, but it was quite a significant change in attitude toward patients. The premise was taken further by the acknowledgment that for patients to participate with their physicians in deciding whether to use birth control pills, there needed to be a source of information. And there was the further acknowledgment that perhaps doctors were not going to delineate all of the options women had and that written materials might be useful. Finally, there was the desire on the part of many to be sure that women knew the side effects of birth control pills so they could make a truly informed choice. All of this sounds like a given today, but it was not just 20 years ago. Twenty years ago, this was regarded as forward, indeed revolutionary, thinking.

I remember sitting at the FDA with the people assigned to draft the first PPI for birth control pills and trying to think through with them what kind of information was appropriate and what was not, how much information was too much, and how to simplify the language so that even a ninth grader–or a fifth grader perhaps–could understand it. With all the published books today containing consumer information about prescription drugs, it appears to be easy to draft patient information, but the reality is that the early efforts entailed considerable debate.

The PPI for OCs proved successful. It notified women of the serious risks of OCs. It did not cause a major disruption in the doctor-patient relationship. It did not change the product liability situation. It did not diminish the role of the pharmacist in patient counseling. All of the dire predictions did not come true. So, for the remainder of the 1970s, there was continued use of PPIs to communicate information about prescription drugs.

At the same time that PPIs were becoming more accepted, other trends were beginning to take shape. Pharmaceutical companies recognized that consumers were more interested in information about prescription products and were becoming more active in making therapeutic decisions with their physicians. This led companies to focus their own attention on providing such information to the public.

In the late 1970s and early 1980s, there was the beginning of the kinds of health care communications techniques that we see today: more press releases issued by pharmaceutical companies to keep the public informed about new drugs and ongoing research; the development of video news releases (VNRs)–video versions of written press releases–so that television stations can have equal access to stories in a format they can use; backgrounding sessions for medical reporters so that the media can write more knowledgeably about new therapies; and the sponsorship of media tours by drug companies, in which physicians or other health professionals are placed on radio or TV shows to discuss a particular disease or treatments.

It is also important to note that Wall Street's interest in drugs also began to influence the information that drug companies issue. Wall Street analysts have become the new public gurus of medical technology. They are quoted in the media more frequently than physicians when new drugs are approved. Actually, this is fortunate because in many cases they know more than physicians do at this stage. Thus, the public's first exposure to the value of new drugs often comes from people who are more accustomed to reading balance sheets than medical records.

Let me move on to relate from personal experience how the FDA's own position on the issuance of information about prescription drugs changed in this period. Until 1978, the position of the agency was that it would never announce the approval of a new drug. The thinking was that a government announcement would imply endorsement of the product. Further, the thinking was that it was the responsibility of drug companies to announce and promote their own products.

In 1978, the agency was under considerable pressure from epilepsy groups to approve sodium valproate, a drug for epilepsy that was available overseas. The drug became a cause célèbre, and resulted in media attention. The FDA took the unusual step of aggressively seeking the data on the drug and actually helping to put together the new drug application. When the FDA was about to approve it (more quickly than even the sponsoring company had anticipated, I might add), the decision was made to issue a press release. It seemed the logical thing to do in view of the external pressure.

The reaction was major stories in the news media that made the FDA look very good. That happened to be at a time when the FDA was accused of causing a drug lag in the United States; that is, delaying through bureaucratic inertia the approval of new drugs that were available earlier overseas. The sodium valproate coverage showed that the FDA did indeed approve some drugs and could do so quickly. The decision was made from very high in the Department of Health, Education, and Welfare that the FDA should continue to announce selective new drug approvals.

Ironically, from a policy of never announcing drug approvals, the FDA and the government health establishment have gone to the other extreme. Announcements of new drug approvals and of new research findings emanate from the government virtually every week. Not only the FDA, but also the National Institutes of Health issue such announcements, as do the major medical journals. It sometimes appears that the government and medical journals are falling all over themselves to announce their own latest accomplishments, a point that should not be lost as we consider the role of pharmaceutical companies in providing similar information to the public and the media.

I want to pick up in my discussion of the history of consumer communications about prescription drugs by mentioning direct-to-consumer advertising. In 1981, the Commissioner of the FDA, Dr. Arthur Hull Hayes, Jr., said in a speech that he anticipated efforts in the 1980s to advertise prescription products directly to the public. The industry interpreted this as meaning that the FDA would not stand in the way of such communications. It was never Dr. Hayes's intention to unleash a barrage of direct-to-consumer ads, but his remarks threatened to do just that, and they led to a request by the agency for a voluntary moratorium on such advertising. The moratorium was lifted in 1985, and the FDA said that the same standards that apply to prescription drug advertising to physicians would apply to prescription drug advertising to consumers. Since then, there has been considerable experimentation with direct-to-consumer advertising, both in print and on television.

The print ads have been of two varieties: (1) the general health message, in which the advertiser helps educate the consumer about a disease, suggests there may be treatments that can help, and urges a visit to the physician and (2) product-specific ads, which we are now seeing with increased frequency. These latter must meet all of the standards for prescription drug advertising, including fair balance and full disclosure via the brief summary that appears in very small type, usually on the page following the ad. The TV ads, generally speaking, have been only of the health message type. These are ads that identify a disease and urge a visit to the doctor. There have been a few product-specific TV ads–for Rogaine® and Nicorette®, for example–but to comply with FDA regulations, these ads cannot say what the drug is used to treat.

The advertising that is now taking place on television is quite restrictive because of the FDA's insistence that such advertising meet all the requirements of the regulations. This means that if the name of the drug is mentioned, along with its use or indications, there must be full disclosure in the form of the brief summary. No one has yet figured a way to reasonably have full disclosure within the confines of the TV screen.

The FDA has made special accommodation for product-specific ads that make medical claims and that are directed at physicians on Lifetime Medical Television. The special provisions require a crawl of the package insert, which can occur at some time other than when the ad appears, and the provision of an 800 number for complete prescribing information. But, in general, the FDA's insistence that TV advertising meet the full disclosure requirements has precluded significant advertising of prescription drugs on television.

There are a number of considerations that will drive the future of health care communications. First, there are no signs of any diminished interest by consumers or by the media in health care information. If you look in the bookstores, watch television, or talk with your neighbors, you can readily see that people are interested in health care information. I hope we can stipulate that consumer interest in health issues will remain strong and, in view of the aging of the population, very likely intensify.

One of my associates at Burson-Marsteller, who is watching the development of health care communications from afar, believes that the broadening of avenues for communicating health care information is inevitable, regardless of the FDA or congressional constraints, simply because the public will continue to demand such information, and that demand will drive the issue. In any event, consumers definitely want to make informed choices about their own health care, including the selection of drugs, and they will need information on which to base those choices.

Second–and again I have no scientific data to support this, but I hope we can stipulate it–I believe that at least some patients are not satisfied with the way that their physicians communicate information to them. If consumers were satisfied, then they would not be buying all of these books, including the *PDR*. In addition, there are changes in how patients relate to doctors. With HMOs becoming more common, the traditional relationship between patient and family physician is altered. Further, with people moving their homes so frequently, there are fewer people with doctors who know their complete medical histories. So, there is a continued demand for information about health, and there remain gaps in the present means of communicating this information from health care professionals. What this means, in essence, is that there is a vacuum of information to be filled.

If there is such a vacuum of information sources, who is available to fill them? There are many sources. As I mentioned before, the government certainly has not been silent during this revolution in the demand for health care information. The FDA, the National Institutes of Health, and the Centers for Disease Control all spend millions of dollars in issuing information to the consumer. Indeed, when I hear criticism of issuing health care information with video news releases, I note in response that the government issues VNRs to help television reporters cover its stories.

There are other sources as well. As I mentioned before, the *Journal of the American Medical Association* and the *New England Journal of Medicine*, arguably the two most reputable and widely quoted medical journals, both issue news releases every single week announcing the latest studies they are publishing. These releases are clearly targeted toward a consumer population.

Another resource for consumers about health care information is printed material, books, magazines, and newspapers. The bookstores and magazine racks are filled with such publications. Close to 75 daily newspapers now have health sections catering to those seeking such information. Some of the printed information is reliable, some is not. Some focus on new products, others focus on relationships with health professionals. Some even give medical advice based on consumer letters.

Still other sources of medical information for consumers are the TV talk shows–Donahue, Oprah Winfrey, Geraldo Rivera–and what I call the entertainment shows disguised as news shows, shows like Sixty Minutes,

Prime Time Live, and 20/20. These shows are constantly doing segments on health care themes, usually from the negative perspective. In the same vein, there are many talk shows just about medicine. In Washington, for example, Dr. Gabe Mirkin dispenses medical advice via the radio.

Another source of medical information for consumers is congressional hearings. These hearings, focused on a single issue, are played to and for the media and often receive huge amounts of media attention, not just on the day of the hearing, but sometimes for months afterward. Knowing the old saying that "There ain't no news in harmony," those who set up these hearings are focused on controversy, wrongdoing, and emotion. The witnesses at such hearings are sometimes plaintiffs in litigation or their lawyers, who use the hearing for their own purposes. Sometimes they are dissident employees who disagree with the decisions of their employers, be they the government or private industry. Sometimes they are government decision makers whose judgments are second-guessed, or they are company representatives who defend their actions. Congressional hearings are conducted in theatrical settings that hardly represent scientific exchange.

Finally, we come to the manufacturers of products. They, too, via the means I have already described, such as press releases, are the sources of much medical information for consumers. While some of the information they issue is designed to be strictly educational in nature, it is neither a secret nor a surprise that the vast majority is ultimately intended to market a product. But such marketing efforts also play an essential informational and educational role as well.

It may be worthwhile to note the one major distinction between all these other sources of information and the pharmaceutical industry. Unlike the statements made by government agencies, medical journals, media, TV and radio talk shows, congressmen at hearings, plaintiffs' lawyers, or dissident employees, the statements made by pharmaceutical companies, or anyone associated with them, are strictly regulated. They, and only they, are required to be accurate and fairly balanced. In any event, the point I want to make is that the information gap that exists between consumer demand and the ability of the health professions to provide that information is being filled by many, many sources.

My next point relates to what I see occurring in health care communications. I will start with the health care environment as it affects the pharmaceutical company. What I see is a very competitive marketplace, with many companies often competing for the same prescribing physician. I see the development of new consumer-driven drugs–for cholesterol lowering, arthritis, birth control, and the like–where consumer information and education is of special importance. I see continued strong pressure on prices, with especially intense pressure from government and other third-party reimbursers. What this all means is that marketing of pharmaceuticals and communication about pharmaceuticals must be and will be aggressive and must also be cost-effective.

What will delay, and perhaps cancel out, the expanded use of new health care consumer communications is what I call the countercurrents, the forces that are arrayed against pharmaceutical information to consumers sponsored by drug companies. The opposition stems from several sources, but these sources have many elements in common. They believe that prescription drugs are different from consumer products and should not be promoted or marketed in the same way. They believe that the kind of information being communicated is of such a complex and fundamentally important nature that it should be communicated on an individual basis, through a health care professional. They believe that generalizations about the safety and effectiveness of a drug are dangerous because drugs can be safe and effective only on an individual basis, depending on an individual diagnosis. And they believe that drug companies cannot be trusted to communicate directly with patients without confusing education with product promotion.

The opponents of expanded consumer communications from pharmaceutical companies include:

- Representative John Dingell, the powerful Chairman of the House Oversight and Investigations Subcommittee. He is skeptical, at best, about direct-to-consumer advertising and has more influence at the FDA than any other congressman.
- Senator Edward Kennedy, Chairman of the Labor and Human Resources Committee in the Senate. He is concerned about the appropriateness of certain promotional and marketing practices and about the extent to which their cost increases the price of drugs.
- The American Medical Association (AMA), which recently issued guidelines establishing new criteria for relationships between drug companies and physicians with respect to gifts, reimbursement for travel to symposia, and other matters. The AMA guidelines were adopted by the Pharmaceutical Manufacturers Association. The AMA guidelines do not deal specifically with promotion, but they do provide new thinking on what the relationship between drug companies and physicians should be.
- The Food and Drug Administration, which for the past decade has been increasingly concerned about company promotional practices,

is now in the midst of what Commissioner Kessler calls a crack-down on misleading promotion. The FDA will be issuing new guidelines on symposia and on direct-to-consumer advertising, guidelines it has promised for several years now. The FDA is also adding new staff to its Advertising Division and has signaled its intention to be more enforcement minded. Dr. Kessler has a special interest in this subject, as he published an article about prescription drug advertising and promotion just before being confirmed as Commissioner. Hopefully, in its zeal to regulate, the FDA will not inhibit the free flow of information to consumers, physicians, or other health professionals.

These are obviously formidable, influential, and powerful forces op-posing expanded consumer communications sponsored by drug compan-ies, especially the FDA's new initiative. In the coming months and years, I believe that the clash of these forces will become one of the most inter-esting and controversial debates, one that potentially goes so far as to in-clude questions of constitutionality under the First Amendment.

Let me make a few brief concluding observations.

It seems to me that one of the fundamental differences between pro-ponents and opponents of expanded consumer communications about pre-scription drugs is a basic philosophical disagreement over the appro-priateness of promoting these products directly to consumers under any circumstances. I know of few physicians, including those who are strongly pro-consumer, who advocate expanding information about pre-scription drugs to consumers, especially information provided by drug companies. Indeed, there are people who believe that prescription drugs should not be marketed at all, that they should merely be available for prescribing. Thus, there are much larger issues here than just policies and regulations. The real issue in many minds is whether there ever is any justification for promotional and marketing activities for prescription drugs. Those who support expanded consumer communications recognize its educational value. Don't consumers have just as much right to learn about new prescription products as physicians and pharmacists? To the extent that pharmaceutical companies are precluded from actively partici-pating in efforts to inform the public, it is likely that less responsible sources may fill the time and space.

One thing is clear, however: if the pharmaceutical industry wants to maintain its strong presence as a source of information, it must demon-strate the educational value of its endeavors. The times seem to call for research on how valuable a commodity marketing and promotional efforts really are.

I think it is ironic that many of the opponents of expanded consumer communications about prescription drugs are individuals who are normally on the side of the consumer and of access to information. One consumer group seems opposed to promotion of prescription drugs directly to consumers, but advocates making available to patients complex information about mortality rates in certain hospitals. In the same vein, the FDA has long stood on the platform that more consumer information is better, yet it takes the view that direct consumer communications about prescription drugs sponsored by drug companies are problematic. These positions seem contradictory and inconsistent, but are not. Rather, they reflect the complexity and underlying philosophical questions posed by the issue of consumer communications about prescription drugs and, perhaps more to the point, a distrust of the pharmaceutical industry.

The same contradictory and inconsistent positions exist at a different level. A speaker at a seminar I recently attended pointed out how ironic it is that cigarettes can be advertised directly to the public with only a brief sentence or two warning, while a prescription product proven to be safe and effective in helping people to stop smoking must meet rigorous full disclosure requirements. How can this inconsistency be justified?

It is very clear that opponents of more consumer communications from drug companies base their concern to a large extent on their lack of confidence in the ability of companies to distinguish between education and product promotion or to contain their enthusiasm over new uses of approved products. The drug industry has few external advocates. For all the contributions that the industry has made to health care, only in recent years has it begun to tell its story and build up a confidence level. But questions remain about the industry's marketing practices, not just to consumers but also to physicians. Unless a higher credibility and confidence level–perhaps trust is a better word–is established, the industry will continue to meet resistance to its efforts to communicate information directly to consumers.

Finally, the issue of prescription drug marketing and promotion is now in the public arena. FDA Commissioner Kessler has placed it there, as has the AMA through the issuance of its guidelines and Senator Kennedy with his hearings. The debate has been going on for years, but there remain fundamental differences of opinion over some issues. How much information do consumers want? What is the best source for information about prescription drugs, other than the physician? What role should the pharmaceutical industry play in the mix? Should the FDA permanently ban, through its regulations, the ability of pharmaceutical companies to provide accurate information to consumers through TV advertising? To what extent should public policy take into account the fact that consumer communication about health care from the drug industry is just a small part of the total exposure of consumers to such information and arguably the most reliable? Are there real First Amendment issues here?

These are the kind of questions that now need debate and resolution. It is commonplace to say that issues are at a crossroads. But this is a time when the cliché happens to be true. At no previous recent time has the issue of consumer communications about health care products been so prominently in the public spotlight. How these issues are resolved will determine for some time to come the future of consumer health care communications.

The Food and Drug Administration's Authority to Regulate Miscellaneous Statements by Pharmaceutical Manufacturers

Richard M. Cooper

Both freedom of speech and the public health are affected by the Food and Drug Administration's (FDA) regulation of statements by pharmaceutical manufacturers about their products. In recent years, this subject has engendered much discussion. Among the topics receiving extensive consideration are advertising of prescription drugs to consumers, promotional practices of pharmaceutical companies, and the First Amendment right of manufacturers to engage in commercial speech (1-10). In addition, the FDA has let it be known that it intends to act more aggressively in enforcing the requirements and prohibitions applicable to drug promotion (11, 12).

A topic that, in my view, has not received adequate attention is the precise nature and scope of the FDA's authority to regulate pharmaceutical manufacturers' statements about their products. With respect to some kinds of statements, the FDA's authority is clear; with respect to others, its authority is subject to serious doubt, doubt that somehow is never reflected in the FDA's own characterizations of its authority. It is the area of doubt that I will consider.[1]

I will use the neutral word "statement" to include any kind of utterance, oral or written, whether by words, pictures, or otherwise. The types of statements I will discuss are miscellaneous statements by manufacturers; that is, statements that do *not* appear in product labels; in official package inserts; in materials that are self-evidently promotional, such as unofficial package inserts, promotional brochures, and point-of-

Richard M. Cooper, J.D., is a Senior Partner at Williams & Connolly, 839 17th Street, NW, Washington, DC 20006.

sale materials; or in advertisements.[2] The kinds of statements I will consider include those in patent applications; filings with the Securities and Exchange Commission (SEC); communications with securities analysts; press releases and other communications with the press; communications with medical and scientific groups through seminars, workshops, journal supplements, and manufacturer-sponsored continuing education programs; testimony at congressional hearings and in judicial and other proceedings; and communications with state agencies.[3-5]

I will focus on three overlapping types of cases that commonly raise issues about the reach of the FDA's authority: (1) cases where the FDA's concern is that the manufacturer has made a statement that is false or misleading, (2) cases where the FDA's concern is that the manufacturer has made an unapproved new drug claim, and (3) cases where the FDA's concern is that the manufacturer has improperly promoted a drug.[6] The legal frameworks for these three types of cases are closely related but different.

THE BASIS OF THE FDA'S AUTHORITY

From time to time, the FDA describes the scope of its authority over manufacturers' statements in very broad and imprecise terms. For example:

> As you know, the FDA is charged under the FD&C Act with assuring that information disseminated by a manufacturer (etc.) which mentions or discusses their [sic] drug product(s) is truthful, accurate, balanced, and consistent with the approved (or permitted) labeling for that product(s). (13)

> [I]f the manufacturer or someone acting as its agent is responsible for the dissemination of the information (reinforced by the fact that they are usually responsible for the generation of the information as well), it falls within the jurisdiction of the FD&C Act and we can and should regulate it. (14)

> Our position is that most company sponsored public relations activities dealing with their product(s) can be considered to be promotional activities (i.e., commercial speech) which are subject to our regulation. (15)

The FDA's view seems to be that, if a statement is made by a manufacturer and refers to the manufacturer's drug, the agency can regulate it. That view reflects a serious misunderstanding of the law.

Under the Federal Food, Drug, and Cosmetic Act (FDCA or 1938 Act), the FDA has four principal, explicit sources of authority over statements by manufacturers (16).[7] First, Section 502(a) makes a drug misbranded if its labeling is false or misleading in any particular (17). Second, Section 502(n) requires that advertising and descriptive printed matter relating to a prescription drug include certain types of information (18). Third, Section 505(b)(1)(F) and (d)(7) give the FDA authority to review proposed labeling in a new drug application to determine whether it is false or misleading. Section 505(d)(1), (2), (4), and (5) require the FDA to determine whether a new drug submitted for approval is safe and effective for use in accordance with its labeling. The entire new drug review process under Section 505 gives the FDA the authority to determine the claims that may be made for a new drug (19, 20).[8] Fourth, Section 505(i) authorizes the FDA to promulgate regulations with respect to investigational use of drugs (21). Section 701(a) gives the FDA power to implement all of these statutory provisions through regulations (22).

False or Misleading Statements. The FDA's authority with respect to false or misleading statements is limited to statements in "labeling," except with respect to prescription drugs, where its authority extends more broadly. The prohibition in Section 502(a), applicable to drugs and devices, is against false or misleading *labeling.* The statutory prohibitions against false or misleading statements relating to a food or a cosmetic are similarly limited (23).

As a practical matter, the FDA's authority over false and misleading statements with respect to prescription drugs extends beyond labeling to advertising and "other descriptive printed matter," although the FDCA does not expressly so provide.[9] Therefore, in determining the scope of the FDA's authority to attack statements as false or misleading, the critical jurisdictional concepts are "labeling," and, with respect to prescription drugs, "advertising" and "other descriptive printed matter." Because the concepts of advertising and other descriptive printed matter do not present particular difficulty, I will focus on labeling.[10]

Unapproved New Drug Claims. The FDA's authority over unapproved new drug claims is not limited to claims made in labeling. Whether an article is a drug depends, generally, on its intended use (24). As I will discuss shortly, intended use may be ascertained from materials that are not labeling, but not from as broad a range of materials as the FDA commonly asserts.

If a statement is an unapproved drug claim, then, with extremely limited exceptions, it makes the product to which it relates an unapproved new drug and therefore illegal (25).[11] Thus, the FDA's power to determine, in the first instance, whether a statement constitutes an unapproved drug claim gives it effective power with respect to manufacturers' statements that might be so construed.

Promotion. The FDA's authority over drug promotion has no explicit basis in the statute. The agency has used its general authorities to prohibit or regulate promotional statements in certain contexts (26). Most importantly, it prohibits promotion of investigational drugs (27).[12] Where the FDA approval of an investigational drug is clearly imminent and the drug is currently available only to investigators conducting clinical trials, questions might well be raised about the authority for and wisdom of a total prohibition of truthful and nonmisleading promotional statements intended to inform the medical community and the public about the drug. In the case of an important new therapy for a serious disease, there may well be significant public benefit in early and widespread awareness of the drug among physicians and patients. Because the prohibition has been in effect for more than 28 years, however, it is unlikely that a court would overturn it now (28).

Although I do not argue that the FDA has no authority to regulate promotion of *investigational* drugs, I do argue that the agency does not have general authority to regulate the promotion of *approved* drugs where the promotion takes a form other than labeling or advertising. I also argue that the FDA's concept of promotion is overbroad.

To develop my argument in logical stages, I will consider the nature of labeling, the sources of relevant evidence of intended use, and, finally, the nature of promotion and the FDA's authority to regulate it.

LABELING

Section 201(m) of the FDCA defined labeling as "all labels and other written, printed, or graphic matter (1) upon any article or any of its containers or wrappers, or (2) accompanying such article" (29). Note the limitation to "written, printed, or graphic matter." There is no textual basis for asserting that oral statements are labeling. The FDA, therefore, has no statutory authority to regulate oral statements (other than those in advertising for prescription drugs) as false or misleading.

To be within the scope of Section 201(m), a statement either must be on a regulated article or its container or wrapper or must accompany the article. In *Kordel v. United States* (1948), the Supreme Court held that to accompany an article, a statement need not physically travel with it, nor even travel at the same time as the article (30). The Court expressly noted that "[i]n this case the drugs and the literature had a common origin and a common destination" (30). It went on to explain, however:

> One article or thing is accompanied by another when it supplements or explains it, in the manner that a committee report of the Congress accompanies a bill. No physical attachment one to the other is necessary. It is the textual relationship that is significant . . . .
>
> The false and misleading literature in the present case was designed for use in the distribution and sale of the drug, and it was so used. The fact that it went in a different mail was wholly irrelevant whether we judge the transaction by purpose or result. And to say that the prior or subsequent shipment of the literature disproves that it "is" misbranded when introduced into commerce within the meaning of § 301(a), is to overlook the integrated nature of the transactions established in this case.[13] (30)

The Court also held that advertising is labeling when it "performs the function of labeling" (30).

There is much here to ponder. The Court conceives of labeling as having a distinctive function: to supplement or explain the product in connection with its distribution and sale. This function is reflected in the textual relationship between the statements and the product.[14] Whether a particular advertisement performs this distinctive function determines whether it is labeling. Advertising for a product that does not supplement or explain it is not labeling.[15] As the Second Circuit has subsequently held in the *Balanced Foods* case, "labeling does not include every writing which bears some relation to the product. There is a line to be drawn, and, if the statutory purpose is to be served, it must be drawn in terms of the function served by the writing" (31).

Moreover, when the distribution of the article and the dissemination of the statements alleged to be labeling are separated in time, the statements are labeling only if the distribution and the dissemination constitute "an integrated transaction," a matter for the fact finder to determine on the basis of competent and admissible evidence.[16] Whether distribution and dissemination constitute an integrated transaction is a function of the temporal and geographic relation between them, the content of the disseminated statements and their relation to the distributed articles, and other factual circumstances.

The Court's analogy to a congressional committee report on a bill is instructive. First, a report is issued by the same committee that reports the bill; and, both formally and in practice, the report is addressed to the members who will consider the bill to which it relates. It therefore has the same intended audience as the bill.[17] The report and the bill thus have "a common origin and a common destination." Second, a report supplements or explains a bill in that it provides information for the use of the audience in taking action with respect to the bill. It may therefore be inferred from the Court's analogy that the distinctive function of labeling (in contrast to the functions of advertising and other statements about products) is to supplement and explain by providing guidance and assistance in the use of a product.

The First Circuit has elaborated on (and, in my view, gone beyond) these notions by holding that "the term 'labeling' must be given a broad meaning to include all literature used in the sale of food and drugs, whether or not it is shipped into interstate commerce along with the article" (32). Even a court adopting a broad definition, however, limits labeling to (1) literature that is (2) used in the sale of a regulated article. The definition excludes oral statements and also excludes written statements that are disseminated outside the context of distribution and sale.

These limitations on the meaning of the term labeling are consistent with the purposes of the statute. As the Second Circuit held in the *Balanced Foods* case in reversing the condemnation of a product:

> It is not disputed that these claims were misleading, but the Federal Food, Drug and Cosmetic Act was not intended to deal generally with misleading claims; much more general proscriptions may be found in §§ 12-15 of the Federal Trade Commission Act, 15 U.S.C. §§ 52-55 (1958). In our view the Food and Drug Act was intended to deal with such claims only when made in immediate connection with sale of the product. (33)

Many of the types of miscellaneous statements with which we are here concerned–patent applications; SEC filings; statements to securities analysts; most types of press releases, press conferences, and interviews; testimony in legislative, administrative, or judicial proceedings; certain communications with state agencies; and certain types of statements to scientific or medical groups–do not fit within this conception of labeling.

Oral statements are excluded. They are not literature.[18]

Patent applications are excluded. They apply to inventions, not to their embodiments in specific products. They also have no connection with the distribution or sale of products, and they are not directed to consumers, prescribers, or other makers of purchasing decisions. Typically, they precede by years the distribution of particular drug products, and they are not part of any integrated transactions that include such distribution. Finally, it would be ludicrous to suggest that firms use patent applications to promote products.

SEC filings and statements to securities analysts are excluded. They, too, are not directed to consumers, prescribers, or other makers of drug purchasing decisions. Typically, they do not supplement or explain products, and they do not guide or assist the use of products. Such statements also have no immediate connection with the sale of products and are not part of an integrated transaction that includes the distribution of products.

Whether statements to the press are labeling depends on circumstances. Oral statements, of course, are not labeling. Written reports by the press of oral statements by a manufacturer also are not labeling because they are not issued by, on behalf of, or under the direction or control of, the manufacturer. An article by a staff reporter in the *New York Times*, even if suggested by a pharmaceutical manufacturer or its public relations firm, is neither labeling nor advertising and is not subject to regulation by the FDA.[19]

Written statements to the press can be labeling if four criteria are met: (1) the statements are issued by, on behalf of, or under the control of a manufacturer, (2) the statements are addressed, immediately or ultimately, to consumers, prescribers, or other makers of purchasing decisions in their capacities as such, (3) the statements perform the function of labeling in that they supplement or explain a product so as to guide or assist in its use, and (4) the statements are immediately connected to the sale of the product to which they refer or are part of an integrated transaction that includes the distribution and sale of that product.[20] These four criteria have general utility in determining whether written statements are labeling.

I would think that many written statements by manufacturers to the press do not satisfy these criteria. If a statement to a trade publication is not communicated by it to makers of purchasing decisions, it fails to meet the second criterion. Even a promotional statement that does not relate with some specificity to product characteristics or performance does not perform the function of labeling and therefore fails to meet the third criterion. Statements in response to unsolicited inquiries from the general press usually lack the necessary immediate connection to distribution and sale and therefore fail to meet the fourth criterion.

The occasions for press releases and press conferences at which specific products are mentioned frequently are not promotional and therefore are not sufficiently related to distribution and sale. Rather, what occasions the manufacturer's statements may be an obligation under the securities laws to make a public disclosure, an attack on a company or its product by a public interest group or a news medium, a strike, or a report of an independent scientific study that relates to the product. These are not promotional contexts. Therefore, I would argue, unless the statements made are blatantly promotional, not fairly related to the context, and satisfy the four criteria just specified, they are not labeling.

Oral testimony in legislative, administrative, or judicial proceedings cannot be labeling. Even written testimony is not in immediate connection with the sale of a product. Moreover, an official proceeding at which testimony is taken is not a promotional context. In many circumstances, such statements fail to satisfy the second, third, and fourth criteria.

Whether communications with state agencies (e.g., regulatory agencies, formulary committees, Medicaid officials) constitute labeling depends on the circumstances of each case. Here also, the four criteria are a useful guide for distinguishing between those statements that are labeling and those that are not. In particular, if the state official who is the recipient of a communication is functioning as a regulator and not as, or on behalf of, an actual or potential purchaser or in connection with an actual or potential purchase (e.g., as reimburser), the communication is not labeling.

Statements by a manufacturer to medical or scientific groups can take a variety of forms, including seminars, workshops, and other types of meetings; medical journal supplements consisting of write-ups of presentations made at such meetings; and pamphlets and brochures reporting the results of studies. Statements in these forms can be labeling if they satisfy the same four criteria; they are not labeling if they do not satisfy them. Again, oral statements are not labeling.

Here, moreover, two complications commonly appear. First, statements in this category generally are not made by a manufacturer or its employees, but by independent third parties having some direct or indirect financial relationship to a manufacturer. These arrangements take many forms. I suggest that the ultimate test is whether the manufacturer exercises sufficient control over the content of the statements that it is fair to say that the statements are *by* the manufacturer. If they are not *by* the manufacturer, they fail to satisfy the first criterion and are not labeling.

Second, statements to scientific or medical groups may be educational rather than promotional; therefore, they lack immediate connection with distribution and sale and for that reason fail to meet the fourth criterion. The FDA has a number of informal rules that address the content of communications to medical or scientific groups at meetings or in journal supplements. The rules require, among other things, that the communications be educational and not promotional, that they be "balanced," that references to unapproved uses be neither frequent nor emphasized, and that the discussion refer to a number of drugs (or other therapies) and not just the product of the sponsoring manufacturer (34-36).

It is important to recognize the limited application of these rules. Their purpose is to separate medical education or scientific exchange from promotion.[21] If statements are promotional, they are connected to the distribution and sale of a product and satisfy the fourth criterion for labeling. Even if this fourth criterion is satisfied, however, a statement is not labeling if it is not issued by, on behalf of, or under the control of, a manufacturer. For example, I would argue that it is not necessary for a manufacturer sponsoring a supplement to a medical journal to demonstrate *both* that it has no control over the editorial content of the supplement *and* that the content is not promotional. A demonstration of *either* condition should defeat a claim that the supplement is labeling. Statements that have the purpose or effect of promoting a product but are not issued by, on behalf of, or under the control of, the manufacturer fail to meet the first criterion and are not labeling.

Even if statements are promotional, satisfy all four criteria, and thus are labeling, these rules do not necessarily determine whether the statements are false or misleading. In some circumstances, statements can be true and not misleading even if they do not, for example, discuss other potentially relevant drugs. Moreover, the affirmative disclosure requirements of § 502(n) do not apply to labeling (37).

RELEVANT EVIDENCE OF INTENDED USE

The intended use of an article can be ascertained from a variety of materials, not limited to labeling. Standard summaries of the relevant law refer to newspaper and magazine advertisements, store placards, television and radio broadcasts, letters, oral representations, speeches, and statements of authorized distributors (38). The Second Circuit has summarized the law as follows:

> In determining whether an article is a "drug" because of an intended therapeutic use, the FDA is not bound by the manufacturer's subjective claims of intent but can find actual therapeutic intent on the basis of objective evidence. [Citation.] Such intent also may be

> derived or inferred from labeling, promotional material, advertising
> and "any other relevant source."[22] (39)

This body of law does not, however, support the proposition that any and
all expressions of a manufacturer's intent are relevant to intended use.

The authoritative interpretation of intended use is found in the legislative history of the 1938 Act. The Senate report on one of the predecessor
bills commented:

> The use to which the product is to be put will determine the category into which it will fall. If it is to be used only as a food it will
> come within the definition of food and none other. If it contains
> nutritive ingredients but is sold for drug use only, as clearly shown
> by the labeling and advertising, it will come within the definition of
> drug, but not that of food. If it is sold to be used both as a food and
> for the prevention or treatment of diseases it would satisfy both
> definitions and be subject to the substantive requirements for both.
> The manufacturer of the article, through his representations in
> connection with its sale, can determine the use to which the article
> is to be put.[23] (40)

The critical point here is that intended use is a matter of the representations made by the manufacturer in connection with sale. The Senate
Report does not refer to any and all representations by the manufacturer;
on the contrary, the report qualifies the reference to "representations"
with the words "in connection with its sale." The intended use of an
article, therefore, is the intended use conveyed in connection with the sale
of the product by the manufacturer to the consumer, prescriber, or other
maker of a purchasing decision. Intended use depends on what the manufacturer communicates to customers in a promotional context, not on
what the manufacturer secretly thinks or on what the manufacturer communicates to nonpurchasers (41).[24]

Patent applications, SEC filings, statements to securities analysts,
testimony in official proceedings, communications with state regulators,
and scientific communications are not communications with customers or
prescribers and are not made in connection with the sale of products.
Therefore, they are not relevant evidence on the issue of intended use any
more than a secret diary kept by the CEO of a manufacturer, stored in his
or her desk, and never disclosed to anyone until discovery in an enforcement action, is relevant evidence. Such materials should not be admissible
evidence on the issue of intended use.[25]

Whether statements to the press are communications to customers and are made in connection with sale depends on the circumstances. The same is true of statements to state agencies and medical or scientific groups.

I would argue that the first, second, and fourth criteria for labeling also apply to statements relevant to intended use. Thus, statements about a product that are not issued by, on behalf of, or under the control of its manufacturer do not establish its intended use, no matter how promotional they may be.[26] Statements not addressed to or calculated to reach purchasers, consumers, prescribers, reimbursers, or other makers of purchasing decisions do not establish intended use, even if they are issued by a manufacturer. And statements that are made in an educational or scientific context, and thus are not made in connection with the sale of the product, do not determine intended use, even if such statements are made by the manufacturer.[27]

Whether a statement to a group of physicians is by, on behalf of, or under the control of, the manufacturer depends on the facts of each case. Among the relevant facts are (1) the contractual arrangements among the sponsoring manufacturer, the organizers and presenters or publishing organization, and any public relations or consulting group involved, (2) how the presenters were selected and other sources of influence by the manufacturer over participants or their presentations (e.g., grants), (3) other indicia of the independence or lack of independence of the participants, and (4) the actual role of the manufacturer's employees with respect to the statements (e.g., any preclearance by them). In my view, mere financial sponsorship by a manufacturer of a presentation (e.g., press conference) by an independent party (e.g., an academic researcher) does not, by itself, make the statements by the independent party statements by the manufacturer, where the manufacturer does not control what is said.[28] Nor, in my view, does a manufacturer become the sponsor of a statement by supplying data or other information or by providing noneditorial services to an investigator at the investigator's request in connection with a presentation by the investigator, where editorial control over the presentation is exercised by the investigator and not by the manufacturer.

Whether a statement is educational or promotional also depends on the facts of each case. Among the relevant facts, in addition to the content of the statement, are (1) the roles, if any, of the manufacturer's marketing and medical/scientific personnel with respect to the statement, (2) the extent to which the statement is subjected to scientific peer review prior to issuance, (3) whether the statement is by a recognized expert, qualified by training and experience to present information as part of a scientific exchange or otherwise to provide education to the particular audience, (4) the context in which the statement is made-e.g., in a seminar room or at a cocktail party, and (5) the nature of the audience and whether the members of the audience paid (or were paid) to receive the statement.[26] Where the identity of the ultimate audience is disputable, the medium of communications used may resolve the matter.

PROMOTION

Promotion, like labeling, must issue ultimately from the manufacturer of the product being promoted. Promotion thus satisfies the first criterion for labeling. Promotion is also addressed ultimately to makers of purchasing decisions and thus satisfies the second criterion. In the discussions of labeling and relevant evidence of intended use, I have argued that promotion connotes a close relation to distribution and sale. In that respect, it also satisfies the fourth criterion.

In other respects, however, the concept of promotion is broader than that of labeling. It is not limited to labeling's distinctive function of explaining or assisting in the use of a product. Moreover, promotion can include oral statements and, indeed, the full range of public relations activities intended to promote a product.

The FDA sometimes forgets, however, that the distinction in 21 C.F.R. § 312.7(a) between promotion and scientific education does not mean that all communications by a manufacturer to the general public are promotional rather than educational. It is worth repeating that the second sentence in the regulation expressly states that the regulation is "not intended to restrict the full exchange of scientific information concerning the drug, including dissemination of scientific findings in . . . lay media." The agency's regulation thus does not seek to restrict the reporting of scientific findings in the general press. To take advantage of this opportunity provided by the regulation, however, a manufacturer would have to confine its statements to the press to "dissemination of scientific findings" and avoid promotional statements that go beyond such dissemination.

Finally, the FDA's authority to regulate promotion is limited to special contexts, the most important of which are investigational drugs, official labeling, and advertising for prescription drugs. Apart from its specific authority to regulate labeling and advertising of approved prescription drugs and to prevent the making of unapproved drug claims, the FDA has no general authority to regulate the promotion of such drugs. Public relations activities and other types of promotion of an approved prescription drug can be carried out free of FDA regulation if they do not constitute false or misleading labeling, if they do not constitute advertising, and if they do not make unapproved drug claims.

OTHER BODIES OF LAW

Thus far in assessing the scope of FDA authority over miscellaneous statements, I have considered only food and drug law. The kinds of statements at issue are also within the ambit of other bodies of law that reflect policies of full disclosure or full discussion. Food and drug law should not be construed or applied so as to restrict such disclosure or discussion unduly.

The patent law encourages full disclosure of patented inventions and their anticipated embodiments in products. The broader the disclosure, the broader the patent protection and the greater the incentive to invent. At a time of questionable American competitiveness in the world economy, preservation of incentives to invent and protection of the full scope of inventions are no small matters.

The securities laws demand full and fair disclosure to the SEC and to the investment community of matters material to investment decisions.

The First Amendment generally protects and encourages, with respect to matters of public interest, discussion that is "uninhibited, robust, and wide-open" (42). Communications with the press and with the medical and scientific communities through means other than promotional labeling and paid advertising are not commercial speech entitled merely to limited protection, but noncommercial speech entitled to full protection. Even commercial speech (if true and not misleading) is entitled to some constitutional protection (1-10).

If the FDA were to seek to regulate or to derive intended use from testimony or other statements in a judicial, congressional, or administrative proceeding, it would engage the countervailing public policies–indeed, in some cases, oaths–that not merely favor, but require, unconstrained truthful speech in those contexts.

In sum, the limitations inherent in the statute on the FDA's authority to regulate miscellaneous statements are reinforced by other bodies of law that govern the contexts in which many of those statements are made and in which the FDA, basically, has little or no business.

NOTES

[1]The general legal principles discussed here also apply to the FDA's regulatory authority with respect to medical devices.

[2]I use the term manufacturer to include a distributor.

[3]In the petitions seeking an assertion of FDA jurisdiction over Premier®, the high-technology cigarette briefly marketed by R. J. Reynolds Tobacco Company, the petitioners urged the FDA to base a determination of intended use in part on statements in a Reynolds patent application. See FDA Docket Nos. 88P-0155/CP; 88P-0155/CP0002 (1988). The FDA declared the matter moot after Reynolds removed the product from the market. Letter from Frank E. Young, Commissioner of Food and Drugs, to Scott D. Ballin, Chairman, Coalition on Smoking or Health (July 31, 1989) (Docket No. 88P-0155/CP). Letter from Frank E. Young, Commissioner of Food and Drugs, to James H. Sammons, Executive Vice President, American Medical Association (July 31, 1989) (Docket No. 88P-0155/CP0002).

[4]For an example of the FDA's reliance on statements in SEC filings to establish intended use, see Regulatory Letter from Daniel L. Michels, Director, Office of Compliance, Center for Drugs and Biologics, to J. Philip Ray, Director, Advanced Tobacco Products (February 9, 1987) (Favor®).

[5]The FDA treated a press kit as labeling in Letter from Kenneth R. Feather to Joseph P. Aterno, (July 13, 1982) (Pfizer, Inc., Feldene®); Regulatory Letter from Jerome A. Halperin to Richard D. Wood (July 27, 1982) (Eli Lilly & Co., Oraflex®).

[6]The FDA also regulates manufacturers' statements to ensure that all required information is included. For my purposes in charting the limits of the FDA's jurisdiction, that category of cases may be disregarded.

New drug cases often include a claim of failure to provide the adequate directions for use required by FDCA § 502(f), 21 U.S.C. § 352(f) (1988), but that claim is ancillary to the agency's assertion that new drug claims have been made. Thus, in this important group of cases that sometimes raise jurisdictional questions, those questions are raised by the new drug issue rather than by the issue of adequate directions for use; therefore, these cases are considered under the second category identified in the text.

The remaining cases involving a concern about inclusion of required information principally involve labeling that is technically deficient. Such cases rarely raise a question of jurisdiction, and I will therefore ignore them.

[7]The statute also gives the FDA authority over various technical aspects of drug labels and labeling. See, for example, § 502(b), (c), (d), (e)(1), (g), (h), (j), (p); 21 U.S.C. § 352(b), (c), (d), (e)(1), (g), (h), (j), (p).

[8]Additionally, § 502(f), 21 U.S.C. § 352(f), makes a drug misbranded if its labeling does not bear adequate directions for use and adequate warnings.

[9]No provision of the FDCA prohibits false or misleading statements in advertising (other than advertising that is also labeling) or expressly authorizes the FDA to prohibit such statements in advertising. On the face of the statute, the

reference to advertising in Section 201(n), 21 U.S.C. § 321(n), has no practical effect.

Section 502(n) of the FDCA, 21 U.S.C. § 352(n), however, mandates certain affirmative disclosures in prescription drug advertising and other "descriptive printed matter" (other than labeling) and authorizes the FDA to require other disclosures in such materials. To this extent, the FDA does have express statutory authority to regulate prescription drug advertising. Moreover, the FDA's express statutory authority to require information in advertising and other descriptive printed matter relating to prescription drugs presumably includes authority to require that the information provided be truthful and not misleading. The agency's disclosure requirements for such materials in effect require truthful, and prohibit false and misleading, statements, either in terms, or by keying statements in such materials to those in approved labeling. See, for example, 21 C.F.R. § 202.1(e) (1990). Section 202.1(e)(6), (7) lists numerous ways in which advertisements are or may be false, lacking in fair balance, or otherwise misleading.

The Federal Trade Commission also has authority to regulate advertising for prescription drugs under Section 12 of the Federal Trade Commission Act (FTCA), 15 U.S.C. § 52 (1988), which prohibits any "false advertisement" of foods, drugs, devices, and cosmetics. Section 15(a)(1) of the FTCA, 15 U.S.C. § 55 (a)(1) (1988), defines the term "false advertisement." Thus, false or misleading statements in prescription drug advertising may be attacked under the FTCA.

Section 502(n) of the FDCA was enacted as § 131 of the Drug Amendments of 1962, Pub. L. No. 87-781, 76 Stat. 780 (1962). The provision was intended to eliminate any overlap between the jurisdiction of the FDA and that of the FTC with respect to the matters covered in § 502(n), S. Rep. No. 1744, Part 2, 87th Cong., 2d Sess. 9 (1962); H.R. Rep. No. 2464, 87th Cong., 2d Sess. 13-14 (1962). The FTC has no authority under § 502(n). See 44 Fed. Reg. 37,434, 37,438 (June 26, 1979).

The FDA and the FTC have entered into a memorandum of understanding that allocates between them regulatory responsibilities with respect to advertising. See FDA Compliance Policy Guide 7155m.01 (Oct. 1, 1980). The memorandum gives the FDA "primary responsibility with respect to the regulation of the truth or falsity of prescription drug advertising."

[10] The terms "advertisement" and "advertising" are not defined in the FDCA or in the FDA's regulations. One regulation, 21 C.F.R. § 202.1(1)(1) (1990), however, is intended to give a broad scope to the term.

Questions do arise as to whether a particular advertisement relates to a prescription drug (and therefore is subject to the full requirements of § 502(n) and § 202.1) or relates merely to some other subject, such as a manufacturer or a disease. See, for example, Regulatory Letter from Peter H. Rheinstein to E.T. Pratt, Jr. (June 4, 1987) (Pfizer, Inc., "The Pfizer Health Care Series"); Letter from Kenneth R. Feather to John E. Wolleben (Feb. 12, 1987) (same); Letter from Thomas W. Cavanaugh to D. J. Bucceri (Aug. 19, 1985) (Hoechst-Roussel Pharmaceuticals, Inc., Trental®).

[11]The term "new drug" is defined in FDCA § 201(p), 21 U.S.C. 321(p). The requirement for approval of "any new drug" appears in FDCA § 505(a), 21 U.S.C. § 355(a). Introduction into interstate commerce of an unapproved new drug is prohibited by FDCA § 301(d), 21 U.S.C. § 331(d). The FDA's regulations provide that the term "new drug" applies not only to a substance not approved for drug use (or exempted from the approval requirement) at all, but also to a substance approved for one use as a drug (or exempted from the approval requirement for one use) but intended for a second use as a drug. See 21 C.F.R. § 310.3(h)(4) (1990).

[12]See also 21 C.F.R. § 312.7(d)(2)(iii) (1990) (permitting a manufacturer or investigator to charge for an investigational drug for treatment use where, *inter alia*, "the drug is not being commercially promoted or advertised").

It is not clear whether any act prohibited by § 301, 21 U.S.C. § 331, is committed when § 312.7(a) or § 312.7(d)(2)(iii) is violated by a manufacturer. It is not clear, for example, that noncompliance with those provisions technically makes the prior approval of an investigational new drug application (IND) invalid and therefore makes introduction of the investigational drug into interstate commerce a violation of FDCA § 301(d), 21 U.S.C. § 331(d). If no prohibited act is committed, the agency's principal formal remedy against the manufacturer would be termination of the IND pursuant to 21 C.F.R. § 312.44(b)(v) (1990).

[13]See also *United States v. Urbuteit*, 335 U.S. 355, 357 (1948) (where leaflets and devices were shipped separately, leaflets were, nevertheless, labeling because they "explained the usefulness of the device in the diagnosis, treatment, and cure of various diseases" and "it is plain . . . that the movements of machines and leaflets in interstate commerce were a single interrelated activity, not separate or isolated ones"); *United States v. Urbuteit*, 336 U.S. 804, 805 (1949) (*per curiam*) (test for labeling is "whether the leaflets were designed for use with the machine and whether they were so used").

[14]See also *United States v. An Article of Device . . . Diapulse Mfg. Corp.*, 389 F.2d 612, 616 (2d Cir.) ("the essential question is whether the printed material seized with the device supplements or explains the device"), *cert. denied*, 392 U.S. 907 (1968); *United States v. Kaadt*, 171 F.2d 600 (7th Cir. 1948) (printed matter labeling because used in sale of drug and explained the use of the drug); *United States v. Lee*, 131 F.2d 464, 466 (7th Cir. 1942) ("among the usual characteristics of labeling is that of informing a purchaser of the uses of an article to which the labeling relates"); *United States v. 8 Cartons . . . Molasses*, 103 F.Supp. 626, 628 (W.D.N.Y. 1951) (book "associated with the articles . . . in a distribution plan . . . .").

[15]See, for example, *Alberty Food Prods. Co. v. United States*, 185 F.2d 321 (9th Cir. 1950); *United States v. 39 Bags . . . "Elip Tablets . . . ,"* 150 F.Supp. 648, 650 (E.D.N.Y. 1957) (newspaper advertisements as evidence of intended use, even though not labeling). But compare *United States v. Research Laboratories, Inc.*, 126 F.2d 42 (9th Cir.) ("labeling" includes advertising), *cert. denied*, 317 U.S. 656 (1942).

[16]See also *Founding Church of Scientology v. United States*, 409 F.2d 1146,

1157-58 (D.C. Cir.), *cert. denied*, 396 U.S. 963 (1969); *United States v. Guardian Chem. Corp.*, 410 F.2d 157 (2d Cir. 1969). In *McNeilab v. Heckler*, C.A. No. 84-1617, 1985-86 FDCA Jud. Rec. (FDLI) 245, 247, 250 (D.D.C. June 5, 1985), the court commented:

> . . . the FDA's authority to regulate labeling does not extend to the print or television advertisements over which plaintiff contends defendants attempted to exercise control. FDA's authority to control labeling extends only to "literature" which "supplements" a drug's package label and which is "distributed to consumers as part of an integrated distribution program" and "constitutes an essential supplement to the label attached to the package containing the drug although this literature may have been shipped separately and at a different time than the drug." See *Kordel v. United States*, 335 U.S. 345, 349-50 (1948); *Alberty Food Products Co. v. United States*, 185 F.2d 321, 324-25 (9th Cir. 1950). This court cannot conclude that newspaper or television advertisements "accompany" intervenors' products or are "distributed" by retailers to ultimate purchasers of the drug as part of an "integrated distribution program." See *Alberty Food*, 185 F.2d at 325; see also *United States v. 24 Bottles "Sterling Vinegar & Honey Aged in Wood Cider Blended with Finest Honey Contents 1 Pint Product of Sterling Cider Co., Inc. Sterling, Mass.,"* 338 F.2d 157, 158-59 (2d Cir. 1964) . . . . The FDA has no authority to act as "advertising czar" over consumer drug advertising . . . .

[17]The interest of courts, lawyers, and others in a committee report is derivative of the fact that the report's intended audience is the members.

[18]In Notice of Adverse Findings from Kenneth R. Feather to Robert P. Luciano (Jan. 27, 1989) (Schering-Plough Corp., Theo-Dur®) the FDA asserted: "Promotional presentations in the form of press kits, media appearances, seminar presentations or publications sponsored solely by a firm are subject to Agency jurisdiction as labeling under Section 201(m) of the [FDCA], or as advertisements under Section 502(n) . . . ." To the extent that assertion applies to oral presentations that are not advertisements, it misstates the law.

[19]But see 44 Fed. Reg. 37,434, 37,438 (June 26, 1979) ("Articles in newspapers and lay periodicals that are supported or influenced by pharmaceutical manufacturers and, therefore, constitute labeling or advertising for a drug are subject to close scrutiny by both FDA and FTC."). If by "supported or influenced" the FDA means something beyond statements that are paid for or controlled by the manufacturer, its position is subject to serious doubt on both statutory and constitutional grounds. A manufacturer might be said to influence a newspaper article simply by responding orally to a reporter's spontaneous questions. In that kind of case, "close scrutiny" by the FDA or the FTC would appear to be unauthorized, and regulatory action directed against either the manufacturer or the newspaper would probably violate the First Amendment. The FDA apparently agrees, at least in part:

Printed matter issued or caused to be issued by the manufacturer or distributor of a drug may not be false or misleading. The Commissioner concludes, however, that FDA does not have authority to regulate articles about specific drugs in newspapers and lay periodicals, other than those that constitute labeling or advertisements, and that any attempt to regulate such articles would raise substantial constitutional questions.

Although the point is not entirely clear, presumably a manufacturer does not "cause" a newspaper to issue an article containing particular statements merely by making the statements to a reporter. In this context, I would argue, control is a necessary element of "cause."

[20]But see Letter from Jerome A. Halperin to John M. Holt (Nov. 19, 1982) (Eli Lilly & Co., Oraflex), where the FDA asserted that 21 C.F.R. § 202.1(1)(2) does not require an intended audience of health care professionals. The FDA reasoned, however, that extensive distribution to the medical press "cannot but suggest an intent that the material be disseminated specifically to the health professions." The agency thus appeared to think it necessary to find that the material ultimately would reach health care professionals.

[21]21 C.F.R. § 312.7(a) (1990), adopted in 52 Fed. Reg. 8798, 8833 (Mar. 19, 1987) provides:

A sponsor or investigator, or any person acting on behalf of a sponsor or investigator, shall not represent in a promotional context that an investigational new drug is safe or effective for the purposes for which it is under investigation or otherwise promote the drug. This provision is not intended to restrict the full exchange of scientific information concerning the drug, including dissemination of scientific findings in scientific or lay media. Rather, its intent is to restrict promotional claims of safety or effectiveness of the drug for a use for which it is under investigation and to preclude commercialization of the drug before it is approved for commercial distribution.

[22]See also, for example, *United States v. Hohensee*, 243 F.2d 367, 370 (3d Cir.) (intended use established by "graphic materials distributed and testimony of oral representations to users and prospective users. The latter are no less relevant on the question than the former."), *cert. denied*, 353 U.S. 976 (1957); *United States v. ". . . Toftness Radiation Detector . . . ,"* Nos. 75-C-478, 75-C-479 (W.D.), 1983-84 FDCA Jud. Rec. (FDLI) 213, 217 (W.D. Wis. Jan. 18, 1983) (intended use of product is determined "from the various circumstances surrounding its distribution"), *aff'd*, C.A. No. 833-1404, 1983-84 FDCA Jud. Rec. (FDLI) 329 (7th Cir. Apr. 4, 1984).

[23]This passage has been cited as authoritative. See, for example, *United States v. An Article . . . Sudden Change*, 409 F.2d 734, 739 n.3 (2d Cir. 1969); *Action on Smoking & Health v. Harris*, 655 F.2d 236, 239 (D.C. Cir. 1980).

[24]In Letter from William V. Purvis to E. L. Schumann (May 15, 1986) (The Upjohn Co., Rogaine®), the FDA asserted that a press release issued by Upjohn was labeling. In Letter from George H. Ishler to William V. Purvis (May 29, 1986), the company denied the FDA's characterization on the ground, *inter alia*, that the release was issued to communicate with the investment community, not the medical community. In its reply Letter from William V. Purvis to George H. Ishler (June 6, 1986), the FDA stated:

> We disagree with your position that the April 29, 1985 press release is not labeling. The press release was conceived, prepared and disseminated by you on behalf of the Upjohn Company. Further, it discusses the safety and efficacy of Rogaine thereby meeting the definition of labeling. . . . Intended audience is not and never has been part of the determination of what constitutes labeling.

The agency's position does not adequately reflect either the case law relating to "labeling" or the legislative history relating to intended use. A communication solely to the investment community is not labeling and is not evidence of intended use.

[25]In *United States v. 354 Bulk Cartons . . . Trim Reducing-Aid Cigarettes*, 178 F.Supp. 847 (D.N.J. 1959), the principal question was whether cigarettes marketed for weight reduction were new drugs. The court reviewed claims made on the exterior of the cigarettes' package, a display card, a window display streamer, a salesman's catalog sheet addressed to retailers, and radio and television commercials. It then quoted from the claims stated in a patent attached to the manufacturer's answers to interrogatories. The court did not discuss the relevance of the patent, nor in analyzing the issue of the product's intended use did it refer to the patent or to any other particular evidence.

[26]A statement may be "by" a manufacturer if it is initially made by the manufacturer or if it is adopted and disseminated by, on behalf of, or under the control of, the manufacturer. Thus, distribution by a manufacturer of an independently produced article in a medical journal makes the article, as distributed by the manufacturer, labeling. By similar reasoning, it could be argued that where a manufacturer sponsors an independent speaker but the speaker's presentation is determined (even though not dictated) by the manufacturer, the speaker's presentation is "by" the manufacturer. The analogy to the journal article breaks down, however, where the presentation is not fully predetermined. To the extent that the speaker is free to speak his or her own views, the actual statements made by the speaker are the speaker's, not the manufacturer's. The FDA apparently is prepared to take the position that an independent speaker's statements are by a manufacturer where the manufacturer "knows" what the speaker is going to say, even though the speaker is fully qualified to develop his or her own views independently of the manufacturer and has done so and the manufacturer has exercised no control over what the speaker will say. Cf. Notice of Adverse Findings from Kenneth R. Feather to Robert P. Luciano (Jan. 27, 1989) (Schering-Plough

Corp., Theo-Dur). In that circumstance, it is highly questionable whether it is appropriate to attribute the speaker's statements to the manufacturer.

[27]The FDA has stated to a firm: "Your firm may sponsor educational activities that provide for mention of your products, involve discussions of extra-labeled uses, and present data favorable to your products relative to competing products. We have, in practice, not required dissemination of full prescribing information as part of this legitimate exchange of scientific information where the information is presented in a manner that is rigorously truthful, non-promotional, objective, and balanced. If a body of data includes significant evidence favoring competing products, a balanced and objective discussion of that data in an educational context will necessarily require discussion of those advantages of competing products as an integral component of a balanced presentation. This general standard applies to the overall presentation, including content and emphasis, as related both to your firm's products and competing products." Notice of Adverse Findings, from Kenneth R. Feather to Robert P. Luciano (Jan. 27, 1989) (Schering-Plough Corp., Theo-Dur).

[28]The FDA apparently is uncertain about this point. In a case where a manufacturer sponsored a press conference by a university medical researcher, the agency stated: "[I]t is illegal to promote a marketed drug for unapproved indications. While we understand that Dr. Voorhees was at liberty to hold a press conference and/or provide press materials *on his own*, your firm had the option of refusing to sponsor this activity. Your sponsorship could be interpreted as a willful attempt to circumvent sections 502(a) and 502(f) of the [FDCA] and section 505 as defined by 21 C.F.R. 312.7(a), which prohibits promotion of an investigational drug." Letter from Kenneth R. Feather to Russell J. Hume (Mar. 10, 1988) (Ortho Pharmaceutical Corp., Retin-A®) (emphasis in original). If the manufacturer did not control what Dr. Voorhees said, his statements were his own, even if the manufacturer paid for the press conference. The heavy-handed threat in the FDA's letter seems wholly unjustified.

REFERENCES

1. Kessler, Pines. The federal regulation of prescription drug advertising and promotion. JAMA 1990;264:2409.

2. Peck, Rheinstein. FDA regulation of prescription drug advertising. JAMA 1990;264:2424.

3. Wang JC. PR update: FDA hints at new guidelines for drug products. Pharm Exec 1989;9(Sept):80-4.

4. Harris JP. Legal restrictions on food, drug, and cosmetic advertising. Food Drug Cosmetic Law J 1988;43:249-67.

5. Fisher KA. The constitutionality of the Food and Drug Administration's regulation of over-the-counter drug labeling under the commercial free speech doctrine. Food Drug Cosmetic Law J 1985;40:188-220.

6. Loevinger L. Free speech in advertising. Food Drug Cosmetic Law J 1984;39:217-29.

7. McNamara SH. FDA regulation of labeling and the developing law of commercial free speech. Food Drug Cosmetic Law J 1982;37:394-401.

8. Barrett. "The uncharted area"–commercial speech and the First Amendment. Univ Calif Davis Law Rev 1980;13:175.

9. Farber. Commercial speech and First Amendment theory. Northwestern Univ Law Rev 1979;74:372.

10. Stone. Restrictions of speech because of its content: the peculiar case of subject-matter restrictions. Univ Chicago Law Rev 1978;46:81.

11. Anon. Drug advertising regulatory action by FDA appears likely: FDA collecting records on repeat offenders in preparation for setting object lesson. F-D-C Rep 1991;53(7):6.

12. Gladwell. New FDA chief promises crackdown on misleading ads by drug firms. Washington Post 1991 Mar 1:A13(col 1).

13. Feather KR. Unpublished speech.

14. Feather KR. Unpublished speech.

15. Feather KR. Unpublished speech.

16. 21 U.S.C. §§ 301-93 (1988). The relevant provisions of the FDCA are §§ 201, 301, 502, and 505, 21 U.S.C. §§ 321, 331, 352, and 355.

17. 21 U.S.C. § 352(a).

18. 21 U.S.C. § 352(n).

19. 21 U.S.C. § 355(b)(1)(F), (d)(7).

20. 21 U.S.C. § 355(d)(1), (2), (4), (5).

21. 21 U.S.C. § 355(i).

22. 21 U.S.C. § 371(a).

23. See §§ 403(a)(1), 602(a), 21 U.S.C. §§ 343(a)(1), 362(a).

24. FDCA § 201(g)(1)(B), (C), 21 U.S.C. § 321(g)(1)(B), (C).

25. See the grandfather clauses in FDCA § 201(p)(1), 21 U.S.C. § 321(p)(1); Drug Amendments of 1962, Pub. L. No. 87-781, § 107 (c), 76 Stat. 780, 788-89 (1962).

26. See 21 C.F.R. §§ 200.7, 200.200, 201.100(f), 201.200(b)(1), 201.200 (e)(3), 201.200(f)(2), 201.56(b) (1990).

27. 21 C.F.R. § 312.7(a) (1990).

28. See 28 Fed. Reg. 179, 180 (Jan. 8, 1963).

29. 21 U.S.C. § 321(m). *Accord*, 21 C.F.R. § 1.3(a) (1990). See also 21 C.F.R. § 202.1(1)(2) (1990).

30. 335 U.S. 345 (1948).

31. *United States v. An Undetermined Number of Cases . . . Balanced Foods, Inc.*, 338 F.2d 157, 158-59 (2d Cir. 1964).

32. *V. E. Irons, Inc. v. United States*, 244 F.2d 34, 39 (1st Cir.), *cert. denied*, 354 U.S. 923 (1957).

33. See the *Sterling* case in Note 15.

34. Kaplan A, Becker R. Labeling or scientific exchange? Pharm Exec 1987; 7(Jan):56-8.

35. Feather KR. Unpublished speech.

36. Feather KR. Unpublished speech.

37. See 44 Fed. Reg. 37,434, 37,437 (June 26, 1979) ("section 502(n) of the act applies only to prescription drug advertising and not to labeling").

38. See, for example, *United States v. An Article of Drug . . . Disotate,* [1976-77 Transfer Binder], Food Drug Cosmetic Law Rep (CCH) Par. 38,086 at 38,287, 1975-76 FDCA Jud. Rec. (FDLI) at 239, 241 (E.D. La. Sept. 28, 1976).

39. *National Nutritional Foods Association v. Mathews,* 557 F.2d 325, 334 (2d Cir. 1977) (citations omitted).

40. S. Rep. No. 361, 74th Cong., 1st Sess. 4 (1935) (explaining definitions in S.5, which, in relevant respects, are substantially the same as those in the law as later enacted).

41. The objective nature of "intended use" is reflected in 21 C.F.R. §§ 201.128, 801.4 (1990), although those regulations go beyond the decided cases.

42. The phrase appears in *New York Times Co. v. Sullivan,* 376 U.S. 254, 270 (1964), which applied to speech about government affairs.

The Benefits
of Pharmaceutical Promotion:
An Economic and Health Perspective

Alison Keith

Promotion conveys information, and information makes markets work better. In the context of prescription drugs, the benefits of promotion are better health and more vigorous competition, which, in turn, put downward pressure on prices.

The most direct informational effect of promotion, and the one easiest to see, is that it helps people sort through the array of available goods and services to choose those best suited to their needs and preferences, within the always-present constraint of ability to pay. With prescription pharmaceuticals, better information makes better matches of patients with drugs possible, leading to improvements in health (1).[1]

Promotion has indirect effects as well–powerful effects. It enhances competition, putting downward pressure on prices. It makes it easier for new products to attract buyers and is, therefore, an incentive for innovation. By facilitating the entry of new products and new firms, promotion further strengthens competition on quality and price.

This view of promotion is not unanimous, of course, yet whether promotion adds or subtracts from the well-being of society is less controversial among economists than among other observers. For example, many critics of promotion allege proliferation of misleading messages. Many economists respond that even without taking government regulation into account, it is highly unlikely that most promotion would be misleading. Firms planning to stay in business for the long term have strong disincentives against misleading buyers; it is simply too costly to lose and then rebuild a good reputation. Moreover, modern economic theory

Alison Keith, Ph.D., is Assistant Director for Economic Analysis, Pfizer Incorporated, Pharmaceuticals Group, 235 East 42nd Street, New York, NY 10017.

emphasizes the importance of information in causing markets to perform well, and at the same time, generating and disseminating information is costly. Promotion is seen as a potentially valuable means of helping buyers make choices tailored to their preferences. Promotion is not dismissed as useful only to profit-hungry sellers. The debate among economists focuses instead on questions such as whether there is too much promotion and whether promotion by established firms hinders the entry of new firms.

In this paper, I will explain the economic logic linking promotion with direct and indirect benefits. I will report the results of some economic studies of the effects of promotion in pharmaceutical markets and studies on some other markets as well. Finally, I will develop the implications for public policy of the view that promotion is valuable in making markets work better. Specifically, I argue that overrestrictive regulation of promotion can harm consumers by preventing them from getting useful information.

PROMOTION AIDS MATCHING
OF PATIENTS WITH DRUGS

It is easy to list a number of dimensions, such as indications and contraindications, on which a physician must have information to match a patient with a drug. Similarly, information on differences in side-effect profiles for therapeutic alternatives allows doctors and their patients to evaluate which side effects are clinically most important, which are most likely to influence compliance, and which the patient will find least distasteful. Another element of a good match is matching value to price. Many consumers still pay much of their prescription drug bills out of their own pockets. Some may be willing to accept some inconvenience or bad taste or even an unpleasant but nonthreatening side effect if the price is lower, while others are willing to pay more for what they view as a better drug. Only with sufficient information can physicians working with their patients make the best choices among therapeutic alternatives, and more precise prescribing decisions translate into better health outcomes.

It is abundantly clear, then, that information is critical to the best use of prescription drugs. Indeed, the most useful way to view a prescription product may not be as a tablet or an ointment standing alone, but as a composite, the physical product bonded with the information. Consider the physical product in isolation, stripped of information about it. If physicians were simply handed a pharmaceutical product without information on what it could accomplish and how it should be used, they would be at sea as to when and how to prescribe the product.

This situation is not entirely fanciful. In some less developed countries, where intellectual property rights are not acknowledged in the same way as in the U.S., generic products are sometimes approved even before the originator's product is approved. For example, Pfizer, the company that developed the antiarthritic Feldene® (piroxicam), was not the first company approved to sell piroxicam in Turkey. Another company, after obtaining first marketing rights, sold piroxicam without educating physicians about its use, perhaps because without being intimately involved in the development and testing of the drug, the company did not have sufficient information about it. Sales of the product were initially modest, then declined, even while Feldene was finding widespread acceptance in other countries. Later, when Pfizer also obtained approval to market Feldene in Turkey, it found the task of educating physicians about the drug more difficult because it had to overcome the negative attitudes toward piroxicam that physicians had developed when they had tried the drug without adequate understanding.

Indeed, information is formally the linchpin of the Food and Drug Administration's (FDA) entire regulatory system. A product is not simply deemed acceptable or unacceptable per se. Rather, it is approved for certain indications with specific directions for use. Only after the approval of the information–the information that makes the product useful–is a company allowed to market a new product.

While there can be no doubt that information is valuable, it is costly to produce and disseminate information. Promotion can be analyzed as to its cost-effectiveness as a way of getting information to the person who makes the decision. I focus on promotion to physicians, since it is the physician who has the authority to prescribe.

One way for information to get into the prescribing process is for each physician independently to seek new information about prescription drugs by reading journals and consulting with professional colleagues. Economists speak of this process as "search." Search is not costless. The most costly component is typically time. The value of the time spent in search is measured by the value foregone, the value of the time had it been spent doing something else. For a physician, seeing patients is a high-value alternative use of the time spent in search. In light of the high opportunity cost of their time, physicians may find they cannot afford to spend many hours in searching out information on prescription drugs.

If self-initiated search is too expensive, the total amount of information physicians gather is likely to be less than if there is another, cheaper way for the information to reach them. One alternative method is through pharmaceutical companies' representatives, who visit doctors' offices to explain new evidence about disease processes, new therapeutic approaches, and new information about old products. If these representatives make it easier for doctors to receive information, doctors are likely to get more information and, therefore, to be in a position to make even better prescribing decisions. This second information-dissemination technology may be cheaper than the first–cheaper for the doctor but perhaps cheaper also for society as a whole–in terms of total resources needed to effect the transfer of information, including the doctor's time. If this information delivery technology is indeed cheaper, it is likely to be used more, and more information will reach physicians.

If promotion were to do nothing but speed up the dissemination of information, it would benefit consumers. It is plausible that without company-generated promotion, doctors would eventually learn about a new product by reading about the new drug's approval in FDA publications or newspapers and by word of mouth. With promotion, however, more doctors hear about it quickly and start using the new product sooner, and more patients receive superior therapy right away. By generating appropriate use of the drug more rapidly, promotion provides health benefits.

EVIDENCE ON HEALTH EFFECTS OF PROMOTION

The logic that promotion fosters health is upheld by statistical evidence. Even advertising severely attacked by critics has nevertheless had impressive health-promoting effects. Two examples, described below, are health claims for food and advertising for cigarettes. Evidence from a public service campaign provides a first example.

Television Advertising About Colon Cancer Risks

A four-market public service advertising program was recently conducted by the Advertising Research Foundation for the Advertising Council (2). A single advertisement with the message that people should ask their doctors about colon cancer was shown over the period of one year. In the four viewing areas, the proportion of men aware of the usefulness of consulting a doctor about colon cancer jumped from about 6% to over 30% by the end of the year, and the number of men who did ask their doctors rose by more than 75%. The sponsors estimated that if the single commercial had been shown nationally, it would have persuaded 1.7

million to 2.7 million men over the age of 40 to consult physicians about colon cancer.

These television commercials clearly brought about substantial changes in health-seeking behavior. They happened to be public service messages, but information on the risk of colon cancer was also provided by producers trying to sell their own products.

Fiber Claims for Ready-to-Eat Cereal

Commercial messages highlighting the link between fiber and colon cancer, combined with emphasizing the fiber content of individual ready-to-eat cereals, led to increased fiber consumption through cereals and to the introduction of new high-fiber cereals. This began in 1984, when Kellogg began to promote its All-Bran® cereal as high in fiber. With the cooperation of the National Cancer Institute, Kellogg also emphasized the link between increased fiber consumption and a lower risk of colon cancer. Other companies followed Kellogg's lead in emphasizing fiber content.

Ippolito and Mathios studied the effect of these health claims in the ready-to-eat cereal market (3). Using survey data on actual food consumption, along with data on the composition of individual products, they showed that consumers changed their behavior and that advertising was an important source of information. The link between fiber and a reduced risk of colon cancer was known before 1984, and that information was available through government publications and the media. Yet the introduction of advertising made a dramatic difference in people's behavior. Before 1984, there had been no noticeable increase in fiber consumption through ready-to-eat cereals. In contrast, in the 3 years after Kellogg first introduced its health claim, the weighted average fiber content of cereals actually consumed rose by 7%.[2]

Producer health claims also led to significant product innovation. New cereals introduced in the advertising period were significantly higher in fiber (2.59 grams per ounce) than either the average cereal available prior to the advertising period (1.56 grams) or the new cereals introduced between 1978 and 1984 (1.70 grams) (3).

Cigarette Advertising Led to Lower Tar Cigarettes

As a second example, cigarette advertising–perhaps even more controversial than health claims–also led to changes that were beneficial to health. Cigarette advertising does more than affect the number of cigarettes sold.[3] In particular, just as with ready-to-eat cereals, it changed the mix of cigarettes bought and the nature of products introduced into the market.

In the 1950s, there was a surge of advertising that featured tar and nicotine claims, termed the "tar derby." During that same time, and seemingly at least in part as a result of the tar derby, the average tar content of filter cigarettes declined by approximately 31% between 1957 and 1960, due in large part to the introduction of new products lower in tar (4). In turn, later epidemiological evidence has shown that low-tar cigarettes have been a significant factor in reducing deaths from lung cancer. There was also a roughly 40% reduction in nicotine between 1956 and 1960, despite the fact that experts were saying, as late as 1951, that such reductions were impossible from a technical point of view.

The rapid rate of improvement in the health characteristics of cigarettes–that is, in making them less unhealthy–slowed after 1960, when tar and nicotine claims were banned from advertising. In 1960, the Federal Trade Commission negotiated a voluntary agreement with the industry that eliminated all tar and nicotine claims in cigarette advertising because the agency believed there was no precise means of measuring tar and nicotine content.[4] The inability to make tar and nicotine claims reduced the incentive to make product changes by eliminating the opportunity to attract buyers by featuring lower tar.

PROMOTION'S ECONOMIC EFFECTS: ENTRY, PRICES, AND INNOVATION

Promotion not only facilitates healthier behavior and encourages the introduction of healthier products but also powerfully affects more traditional economic measures of a market's performance: prices and the pace of innovation. The controversy over whether promotion improves or worsens the performance of markets–any market, not just the market for pharmaceutical products–has been vigorous. Although the controversy is not fully resolved, there is convincing evidence for the hypothesis that promotion leads to lower prices. It also strengthens competition by facilitating the entry of new products and new firms.

After summarizing the reasoning associated with two competing hypotheses, I report the results of some studies on retail advertising. I then describe briefly several studies on the effects of promotion by pharmaceutical companies.

Persuasion vs. Information

A shorthand for the controversy is whether advertising is primarily persuasive or primarily informational. Because ease or difficulty of entry by new competitors exerts such a powerful influence on a market, a principal criterion for judging whether promotion is beneficial is whether it facilitates or hinders entry.

The hypothesis that promotion is primarily persuasive is built on the following line of reasoning: Advertising and other forms of promotion create strong brand loyalty. This strong brand loyalty allows sellers to charge higher prices because customers are less willing to switch to another product for any specific price difference. Promotion by established firms also makes it more difficult for new firms to enter the market or for existing firms to introduce new products because customers are more unwilling to switch to an unfamiliar product. Since the existence of more competitors puts downward pressure on prices, the absence of this competitive pressure–and indeed the absence of the threat of entry–keeps prices higher than if there were less promotion. This persuasion argument is associated with the term "barriers to entry," and those who argue or find that promotion erects such barriers infer that advertising is primarily a matter of persuasion.

The second hypothesis, that promotion is primarily informational, is that promotion leads to lower prices by making competition more vigorous. It does this by informing buyers about alternatives. When buyers compare alternatives, they compare on the basis of product characteristics and quality, but they also take price into account. Even if the promotion does not mention price, its effect is to make people consider whether the option to which promotion has directed attention is superior to the familiar choice, given the relative prices and product attributes. Proponents of the information hypothesis also argue that promotion facilitates the entry of new products and new firms. It does this by allowing a new seller to draw attention to the novel characteristics of the offering. New entry and awareness by established firms of the threat of entry put further downward pressure on prices. Research showing that promotion facilitates entry implies that promotion is primarily informational.

I do not pretend to provide in this paper a full review of the many economic studies on these issues. I refer to two types of studies only: first, studies of retail advertising regulations showing that advertising has led to lower prices and, second, three recent studies of promotion by pharmaceutical manufacturers, all directly addressing the persuasion or information question.

Retail Advertising Prohibitions Raise Prices

Several studies on various products and services show that prices fell when advertising was introduced into retail markets. These studies took advantage of the presence of advertising in some states and its absence in other states due to state-to-state differences in regulations about advertising. In some states, advertising of certain services was prohibited, while in other states, advertising was permitted and therefore used. A comparison of these sets of states, with appropriate statistical controls, showed differences in prices. The pioneer study, on optometry, was by Lee Benham (5, 6). In states where price advertising was permitted and in states where only nonprice advertising was permitted, prices for eyeglasses were lower than in states where advertising was prohibited. Other studies of retail markets have shown similar effects, including more recent studies of the market for eyeglasses and also studies of such disparate products as retail gasoline and lawyers' services (7-12). John Cady published a similar study on retail pharmacy in which he found that retail prices of prescription drugs were, on average, 5% lower in states that permitted advertising of various forms (13, 14).

These studies stand in contradiction to those who argue that because advertising is costly, prices must be higher to cover those costs. Advertising was an added cost to retailers, yet prices fell. The reasonable explanation is that as consumers found it easier to identify and locate competing sources of products, they shopped more carefully, and retailers, in turn, found it necessary to lower prices to attract and keep customers.

Studies on Promotion by Pharmaceutical Companies Point to Its Pro-Competition Effect

Several studies have been done specifically on the effect of promotion by pharmaceutical companies. These studies have paid special attention to the effect of promotion on the success of newly introduced products.

In the first of this series of three studies, Leffler found that promotion of drugs already on the market made it more likely that entry of therapeutically important new drugs would be successful (15). He inferred that promotion helps, rather than blocks, entry of new drugs and that this is evidence that promotion is informational. A paper in response by Hurwitz and Caves looked at the impact of promotion by pioneer brands when threatened by generic entry (16). They found that such promotion boosted the ability of pioneer brands to maintain their market shares and fend off generic competition. This led them to conclude that the effect of promotion was, at least in part, persuasion, although they concurred in the paper that promotion was, in part, informational. These same authors, joined by a third author, Whinston, noted that for products whose patents expired during the 1970s and early 1980s, advertising by the pioneer brands dropped off before patent expiration and continued dropping before and after entry by generics (17). They noted that total sales in the chemical entity dropped at the same time that advertising dropped. Based on this, they suggest that the advertising seems to have been for the purpose of expanding the market rather than for making it difficult for new products or firms–in this case, generics–to enter, and thus it protected market share and price.

Taken together, these studies point toward (although do not establish beyond doubt) the following conclusion: Promotion in pharmaceutical markets is informational and enhances competition, including through the entry of new products, which in turn can be expected to impose pricing discipline. The studies do not conclude that advertising is, in effect, anticompetitive, shielding sellers from competition and enabling them to keep their prices propped up.

This is consistent with common sense, which links promotion with innovation and thus with facilitating the entry of new products and new competitors. The evidence on ready-to-eat cereal and cigarette advertising reported above similarly links promotion with the introduction of new products. Advertisers are always looking for a new message to capture the attention of buyers. Looking at it another way, the incentive for innovation is increased, since income from the new product will be higher if diffusion is accelerated by promotion. Companies respond to this opportunity for higher income by investing more in developing and marketing new products. Advertising, then, can spur innovation.

PUBLIC POLICY IMPLICATIONS

The view that promotion, for the most part, does not hinder but rather contributes to the efficient functioning of markets has clear implications for public policy. In particular, the standards used by the FDA to judge the promotion of prescription drugs obviously influence–indeed control–the nature and content of advertising for prescription drugs and thus affect the performance of the market.

Since promotion conveys information, overly cautious standards as to what promotion is permitted can harm consumers by keeping valuable information from reaching purchasers or their agents. Two elements of regulation that can have this effect are, first, too-stringent criteria as to what constitutes deceptive or misleading promotion and second, extensive disclosure requirements.

Decisions about what information should be permitted to be disseminated are not simple.[5] Policymakers and regulators must make decisions based on incomplete information, since scientific evidence is always changing. However, much care and attentiveness to the public good must be exercised, any decision may well become outdated as subsequent studies shift the balance between "probably true" and "probably false," and hindsight is sure to show that some mistakes have been made. Policymakers should take into account the predictability that new information will emerge and that some policy decisions will be revealed as mistakes. There are two types of possible mistakes in regulating information flow:

> Type I: Allowing a message that subsequently turns out to be (most probably) false.
> Type II: Prohibiting a message that subsequently turns out to be (most probably) true.

It is not only misleading messages that harm consumers, but missing information as well.

For prescription pharmaceuticals, the paradigm of harm from inaction is familiar from discussion of the so-called drug lag, a term referring to earlier official approval of drugs abroad than in the U.S. Research in the 1970s emphasized the U.S. drug lag compared with the timing of drug approvals in Europe (18). More recently, people with AIDS and people active in seeking clearance for Alzheimer's treatments have been clamoring for early release of drugs. If approvals of valuable new therapies are unduly delayed, those who need those drugs are kept from that health-improving therapy in the interim. In deciding whether to approve marketing of a new drug, the FDA must balance two types of possible errors: the harm that would be done by a drug that turned out to be unsafe or ineffective versus the harm that would be done if the drug turned out to be safe and effective and people had been deprived of its use for some time. The same dilemma that exists with respect to regulation of the marketing of drugs applies also to the dissemination of information.

My recommendation is very simple: compare the harm from a Type I error, along with the likelihood that the Type I error will occur, with the harm from a Type II error, with its likelihood taken into account. It is necessary to look at the likelihood that the weight of the evidence will shift and show something that seemed probably true to be probably false, or vice versa, as well as the harm that will have occurred if such a shift takes place (19).

Instead, the standard too often appears to overweight Type I errors. Regulators and policymakers appear to focus only on the possible harm from misleading claims while disregarding the chance that further evidence may underscore the validity of the information, information that, if disseminated, would have influenced consumer and marketer choices toward better health. An unbalanced list of criteria can mean that too little information is disseminated, with harmful consequences.

It is understandable, of course, that regulators and policymakers have tended to put more weight on preventing errors of commission rather than errors of omission, since errors of commission tend to be so much more visible. Moreover, as long as promotion is viewed primarily as an unavoidable nuisance, policymakers may not even consider the possibility that (over)restrictive regulation poses any possibility of social harm by suppressing information and its economic consequences. Overrestrictive policies may initially seem innocuous, but they are not.

If, instead, promotion is recognized as a valuable and productive means of disseminating information that in turn enhances competition, encourages innovation, puts downward pressure on prices, and ultimately leads to better health outcomes, then regulatory restrictions do not come free. They are costly, and those potential costs, in public policy terms, should be weighed carefully against the possible costs of errors of commission.

It is not only the standard by which deception is judged or, alternatively, by which substantiation of a claim is found acceptable that makes a difference. The same arguments apply to required disclosures, required presumably to avert deception. Disclosures are costly for the advertiser to include, since they take time or space or both. With a higher cost per advertisement, the advertiser is likely to provide fewer advertisements. If so, the main advertising message reaches fewer people in the target audience. Ironically, then, imposing disclosure requirements may lead to less information being disseminated, not more. If the social value of the original promotion is recognized, any gain from the addition of the disclosure must be weighed against the harm due to diminishing the frequency or reach of the advertising. Imposition of a disclosure requirement may have serious and negative consequences for the quality of purchase decisions.

CONCLUSION

Promotion generally improves the functioning of the market. This is true for pharmaceuticals just as for other products and services. Promotion conveys information, making possible improved matching of patients with drugs. Promotion enhances competition, putting downward pressure on prices, and facilitates entry of new products, thereby encouraging innovation and further strengthening competition.

Regulatory standards, and public policy generally, should take into account this valuable informational function of promotion. Policymakers should weigh the harm done to consumers from suppressing useful information rather than focus too single-mindedly on the prevention of deception.

NOTES

[1]The term promotion is used here in a broad sense and includes such disparate forms of communication as pharmaceutical representatives' discussions with physicians, journal advertising, and health messages directed to consumers.

[2]The products were weighted by market shares.

[3]Indeed, statistical studies of advertising have not demonstrated a large demand-increasing effect. According to F. M. Scherer and David Ross, summarizing a series of studies, "The weight of evidence indicates that the long-run growth attributable to advertising has been modest." (Scherer FM, Ross D. Industrial market structure and economic performance. 3rd ed. Boston: Houghton Mifflin Company, 1990.)

[4]Only a few years earlier, many observers believed that there was no strong evidence that these characteristics even affected health. Calfee quotes from a Federal Trade Commission decision in 1950:

> The record shows . . . that the smoking of cigarettes, including Camel cigarettes [the target of R. J. Reynolds advertisements at issue in the case] in moderation by individuals . . . who are accustomed to smoking and who are in normal good health . . . is not appreciably harmful. (4)

[5]There is no place for deliberate falsity in advertising. If there is clear evidence that a claim is false, it should simply not be allowed.

REFERENCES

1. Masson A, Rubin PH. Matching prescription drugs and consumers. N Engl J Med 1985;313:513-5.

2. Advertising Research Foundation for The Advertising Council. Establishing accountability: a strategic research approach to measuring advertising effectiveness. 1991.

3. Ippolito PM, Mathios AD. Information, advertising and health choices: a study of the cereal market. RAND J Econ 1990;21(Autumn).

4. Calfee JE. The ghost of cigarette advertising past. Regulation 1986; (Nov/Dec).

5. Benham LK. An estimate of the price effects of restrictions on drug price advertising on the price of eyeglasses. J Law Econ 1972;15(Oct).

6. Benham LK, Benham A. Regulating through the professions: a perspective on information control. J Law Econ 1975;18.

7. Kwoka JE Jr. Advertising and the price and quality of optometric services. Am Econ Rev 1984;74(Mar).

8. Bond R, et al. Effects of restrictions on advertising and commercial practice in the professions: the case of optometry. Federal Trade Commission staff report. Washington, DC: Government Printing Office, 1980.

9. Marvel HP. Gasoline price signs and price behavior: comment. Econ Inquiry 1979;17.

10. Maurizi AR. The effect of laws against price advertising: the case of retail gasoline. Western Econ J 1972;10(Sept).

11. Porter WR, Jacobs WW, et al. Report of the staff to the Federal Trade Commission. Improving consumer access to legal services: the case for removing restrictions on truthful advertising. November 1984.

12. Schroeter JR, Smith SL, Cox SR. Advertising and competition in routine legal services markets. J Industrial Econ 1987;36(Sept).

13. Cady JF. An estimate of the price effects of restrictions on drug price advertising. Econ Inquiry 1976;14.

14. Cady JF. A statement to the Federal Trade Commission regarding the proposed rules concerning prescription drug price disclosure. January 1976.

15. Leffler KB. Persuasion or information? The economics of prescription drug advertising. J Law Econ 1981.

16. Hurwitz MA, Caves RE. Persuasion or information? Promotion and the shares of brand name and generic pharmaceuticals. J Law Econ 1988;31(Oct).

17. Caves RE, Whinston MD, Hurwitz MA. Patent expiration, entry, and competition in the U.S. pharmaceutical industry: an exploratory analysis. Unpublished.

18. Lasagna L, Wardell WW. The rate of new drug discovery. Drug development and marketing. Washington, DC: American Enterprise Institute, 1975.

19. Federal Trade Commission. Bureau of Economics. How should health claims for foods be regulated? An economic perspective. Economic Issues Paper. By Calfee JE, Pappalardo JK. September 1989.

The Need for Guidelines About Pharmaceutical Promotions Involving Gifts to Physicians

Mary-Margaret Chren

I and others have been concerned that physicians' interactions with drug companies, especially when these interactions involve gifts to doctors, can present a situation in which we might not always act in our patients' best interests (1). On the surface, there is no blatant breach of conduct. Companies have a right to promote their products, and physicians are free to choose what to prescribe. But influences on prescribing that are independent of drug performance data may be insidious and may represent a worrisome ethical situation.

In discussing doctors, drug companies, and gifts, I will first give some examples of gift interactions between doctors and drug companies. Second, I will review evidence that drug promotions such as these affect physician behavior. I will then begin to address the difficult question of ethical ramifications by examining three predictable but ethically neutral effects of physicians' acceptance of gifts from drug companies. There are financial consequences for patients, there may be changes in the image of the profession, and, most important for me, there is the creation of a gift relationship between the physician and the company with whom he or she interacts. Next, I will discuss the rich anthropology of gifts, which are powerful regulators of human relationships. I will address three ethical repercussions of physicians' acceptance of gifts, including injustice, threats to the physician-patient relationship, and possible effects on physicians'

Mary–Margaret Chren, M.D., is Senior Clinical Instructor, Department of Dermatology, University Hospitals of Cleveland, 2074 Abington Road, Cleveland, OH 44106.

Portions of this presentation appeared in the *Journal of the American Medical Association* (1989;262:3448–51), Copyright 1989, American Medical Association, and in the *Rhode Island Medical Journal* (1991;74:603–10).

attempts to balance altruism and self-interest in their professional lives. I will conclude with some practical guidelines for physicians' behavior.

Doctors' friendly contact with drug companies and detail people starts as early as we learn that Eli Lilly is not a brand of stethoscope. The social and professional interaction between doctors and drug representatives is lubricated by a steady stream of gifts that range from advertising trinkets to items of substantial value. Some are useful enough to fill those annoying voids in life. Who ever has enough briefcase-sized umbrellas? How could we continue the business of seeing patients without the ubiquitous office paraphernalia? In case you doubt how ubiquitous it is, consider these data, published in 1988, about promotional materials in patient care areas of a family medicine training center at the Medical University of South Carolina (2). In the practice suite, there were 5 pens, 36 notepads, 1 drug sample, 55 pamphlets and educational posters, and 43 trinkets (such as pushpins, gadgets, key rings, clocks, calendars, paper clip holders, cups, and bags): a total of 140 pieces of promotional material. This averages out to 4.12 pieces of marketing material per individual patient care area.

Some of the gifts I have received are amusingly idiotic, but some are significant, such as a check for $156 made out to me as a senior resident; an invitation to stay–all expenses paid–for six nights at Loew's L'Enfant Plaza, a Washington hotel; and many textbooks and journals (while a junior resident I received the three-volume set *Textbook of Dermatology* by Arthur Rook, for which the list price is $495). Also, many of the interactions involve food and entertainment. The residents in my department average at least one meal per week at drug company expense.

These gifts and other marketing efforts are expensive. Data released at last fall's meeting of the Senate Labor and Human Resources Committee indicated that drug company expenditures on marketing account for about 15% of their revenues (which topped $32.4 billion in 1989), more than they spend on research and development. This translates to $5 billion, or more than $8,000 per M.D. and osteopath (D.O.) per year, on marketing alone. I have been trying to think of ways to impress upon myself how much money $5 billion is:

- It is about two-thirds of the National Institutes of Health annual budget of $8 billion.
- It is 5-10 times the annual tuition of all medical students at all medical schools in the U.S.
- It would pay the salaries of 50,000 clinical pharmacologists at the assistant professor of medicine level. That is 400 new faculty drug experts per medical school.

Who pays this $5 billion in advertising costs? Patients pay for the marketing of drugs. Two-thirds of visits to physicians yield a prescription, and 75% of prescriptions are paid for out-of-pocket, not by insurers. Drug prices escalated 88% between 1981 and 1988, when general price inflation was 28%.

Why do companies spend these vast amounts of money on marketing to physicians? Companies argue that they are committed to physician education and that they need to let us know about their drugs. I and most observers believe that they spend this money because they take seriously their responsibilities to their shareholders. They spend this money because it sells drugs.

But hard data that physician behavior is influenced by other than drug performance are difficult to gather. Elegant work on this topic has been done by Jerry Avorn, of the Harvard Medical School, on scientific versus commercial sources of influence on physicians' beliefs (3). He studied physician perception and use of cerebral vasodilators and propoxyphene (Darvon®). Both were heavily marketed by the companies as being effective, but controlled studies had shown cerebral vasodilators to be useless and propoxyphene to offer no advantage over aspirin. In a survey of a random sample of 100 M.D.s, internists, and general practitioners in the Boston area, Avorn found that 68% felt that drug advertisements had minimal influence on their prescribing. Most felt that scientific sources were the most important determinants of their behavior. Nonetheless, 71% felt that impaired cerebral blood flow is a major cause of senile dementia, a misconception whose main source was advertisements for the cerebral vasodilators, and 32% actually felt that the cerebral vasodilators were useful in managing confused geriatric patients. Forty-nine percent felt propoxyphene was superior to aspirin for analgesia. The mistaken belief in the efficacy of cerebral vasodilators correlated significantly with the mistaken belief in the superiority of propoxyphene.

Because the commercial and academic sources of information about the drugs were diametrically opposed, the physicians' beliefs about the drugs' efficacy was then a "marker" indicating from which sources their information came. Although the vast majority of doctors see themselves as not being influenced by drug ads or detail people, this study suggested the opposite. *The point is that drug promotions affect physicians' beliefs and perceptions.*

A second study looked at self-reports of commercial influences on physicians' prescribing behavior (4). In this survey, 371 faculty and house staff at 7 midwestern teaching hospitals reported an average of 1.5 brief contacts per month with drug representatives. Twenty-five percent of the faculty and 32% of the residents *reported* changes in practice because of this contact. Independent predictors of change in house staff practice were brief conversations. For faculty, predictors of change in practice were brief or extended conversations and free meals. One has to wonder why free meals were so important to faculty.

So I have discussed the amounts of patient money spent on drug promotions in the U.S. and reviewed available empirical data about possibly worrisome influences on our behavior. But it is too broad of an inductive leap to jump from this to an indictment of gifts as ethically suspect. We need to think in measured, logical steps about this difficult situation, where, as Stephen Goldfinger has said, the temptation is to avoid making ethical distinctions because they are hard to make (5). Let me just outline predictable effects of physicians' acceptance of drug company gifts, independent of any ethical repercussions.

First, gifts cost patients money. As we have seen, prescriptions are a major patient expense, and marketing for these prescriptions adds $5 billion a year to their cost. Furthermore, this expense is often passed on to patients without their consent and often without their explicit knowledge. Unlike other forms of marketing, like ads, many gifts are private and not open to public scrutiny.

Second, our acceptance of gifts from drug companies may change society's perception of our profession. American society has traditionally given physicians great freedom to deal with conflict of interest issues ourselves, without legislation. For example, consider the conflicts inherent in our fee-for-service system of reimbursement, where I advise the patient whether or not to get treated, but often, if I treat, I get more income. Such conflicts are, by and large, not regulated by society but are left to the good judgment of the physician, whom society regards as having the patient's best interests at heart. This view, and, in fact, the faith each patient has in his or her doctor may change if people believe we accept or even solicit gifts from drug companies.

Lastly, the mere acceptance of a gift does more than cost money or hurt the reputation of the profession. All gifts establish a *relationship* between the donor and the recipient, a relationship with vague but real obligations. It is this relationship, the gift relationship, that I think is the source of the most compelling ethical dangers in the interactions between doctors and drug companies. I will develop the idea of the gift relationship before turning to the ethical implications of gifts and what we should do about them.

Webster's dictionary defines a gift as "something voluntarily transferred by one person to another without compensation." This definition includes the key features of the common notion of a gift: that a transfer takes place, that the transfer is voluntary, and that there is no recompense. Thus, on the surface, a gift is not an exchange and is not expected nor is it intended to have any effect beyond the transfer of something from the donor to the recipient.

I would like to suggest that Webster's definition is too narrow, missing the essence of a gift, and that the common notion is wrong. I do not expect to convince you that my suggestion is correct; indeed, quantitative data–the sort with which we are all more comfortable–do not exist on this point, to my knowledge. But I hope you will entertain this suggestion as a reasonable hypothesis.

The suggestion that a gift can be more than it seems is not new. Every culture's mythology includes tales, such as that of the Trojan horse, in which a gift holds the seed of destruction for the recipient. It is no accident that a German word for gift has a double meaning: gift in our sense and poison.

A French social anthropologist, Marcel Mauss, explored the meaning of gifts in different cultures (6). He noted that gifts are used to initiate and maintain relationships–the gift relationship. Among pygmies, for example, gifts of earthen pigments and food were used to produce a friendly feeling between the persons concerned. Lest we think this behavior is limited to other cultures and other peoples, let me remind you that at the annual meeting of the American Academy of Dermatology, the "power lunch" of the movers and shakers is given by a cosmetic company, a modern purveyor of earthen pigments which are still used much as they were in earlier times and by other peoples.

Mauss also observed that gifts entail obligations. The obligations of the recipient of a gift include grateful conduct, grateful use, and reciprocation. Although we in modern society have largely lost sight of the importance of gifts as regulators of human relationships, one can think of examples from daily life of the obligations of the gift relationship. Think of the phrase "much obliged," which we use to mean "thank you." Consider how you would feel if your offer of a gift to a spouse or a friend were rejected with a "no, thanks" or "sorry, I can't use it." Think about the last house staff lunch you attended where the food and drink were provided by a drug company. In many departments, each such occasion is preceded and concluded by the ritual of our chief resident blessing the detail person and his or her employer with our thanks.

Mauss further observed that gifts are rarely spontaneous and often not voluntary. The air of spontaneity in the offer, "My friend, I just happen to have a little something for you" is just that, so much air, when we mean "My friend, I have thought about you long and hard. I offer this gift because of what you mean to me and in light of your likes and needs.'' Nor are gifts at expected times–birthdays, anniversaries, visits, and holidays–fully voluntary.

Finally, it can be dangerous to accept gifts. Not only may the gift be destructive to the recipient, as in the case of the Trojan horse, but gifts can also be more powerful than contracts, which can be fulfilled and discharged. Gifts entail obligations in a continuing relationship. A gift is not only a thing without a price; it is, in fact, priceless. To accept a gift without reciprocating can be to accept another's superiority and to face one's own subordination.

The gift relationship, then, is one of paradox: gifts must be given freely, but they entail an obligation. The giver must not insist on any return, yet a response is required. Gift giving is an act of generosity; however, it also serves the self-interest of the giver.

Ralph Waldo Emerson decried the negative, potentially manipulative side of gifts when he wrote, ''It is not the office of a man to accept gifts. How dare you give them? We wish to be self sustained. We do not quite forgive a giver'' (7).

How might we or our institutions respond to a gift from a drug company or its representative? Almost uniformly with a grateful response, the ''much obliged.'' Outright reciprocation in the form of a gift or conscious changes in our medical practices would be unthinkable to most physicians. But many might establish enduring relationships. All of us have friends who dine, travel, or play golf with the marketing representatives of drug companies. Perhaps most importantly, we may respond by granting access to our time and our minds. We might listen to a sales pitch. We might sponsor or attend an educational conference that otherwise might not have been given, a conference on a topic selected or sponsored by the drug company. We might grant or facilitate access to our students and colleagues.

Does the gift relationship affect doctors? As I noted above, there are few published data on this point. The observational evidence is that gift relationships are promoted at great expense by drug companies . . . and also forbidden. These same companies, like many for-profit concerns, generally prohibit their employees from accepting gifts from business acquaintances. These prohibitions are often most strict for purchasing agents, who determine what products their employer will buy, much as physicians determine what drugs their patients will buy. Although the professionalism and motivation of most physicians may lessen their susceptibility to gifts that influence other purchasing agents, one has to wonder whether physicians are really immune. We need more data on this question of influence. But we must act ethically, as always, before all the data are in hand.

Having discussed the gift relationship in its anthropological context, I will now address its ethical implications with regard to justice, the doctor-patient relationship, and the physician's character. Justice entails the fair allocation of burdens and benefits. The problem is that when we accept gifts from drug companies, patients pay but doctors and, undoubtedly, drug companies benefit. As one of our British colleagues so aptly observed, often ". . . we are being given a meal which many of our patients could not afford but which they would appreciate much more" (8).

It has been argued that disclosure to our patients would make the problem of injustice go away. But one must ask, does disclosure really eliminate injustice arising from the acceptance of gifts? In principle, maybe. If the disclosure is full, if the gift is presented as simply becoming part of the doctor's fee, and if the burden and benefit are fairly allocated, then perhaps injustice is avoided.

In practice, however, the answer is probably not. Full disclosure is not the rule. It is tough to estimate the value of gifts associated with a single patient visit. Would I disclose to all my hypertensive patients that my office supplies were provided by the maker of Verapamil-SR®, to my hypercholesterolemic patients that eight hours of continuing medical education (CME) and a fine meal were provided by the maker of Lovastatin®, and to my bronchitic patients that my Caribbean holiday was at the courtesy of the maker of a new oral cephalosporin? Or would I simply say to each patient that, on average, drug companies' gifts to me would add significantly to the cost of their prescriptions? Thus, full disclosure does not look too attractive. So the first ethical implication is injustice.

The second ethical consideration is the physician-patient relationship. All physicians, I think, and many of our patients consider this a special relationship. At the very least, our role is that of a fiduciary who should act in each patient's best interests. Once a physician-patient relationship is established, nothing other than the patient's best interests should influence our care of the patient. The implication is simple. Insofar as gifts influence a physician to prescribe a drug that is less effective or more expensive than an alternative, they threaten the physician-patient relationship. Although the extent of that threat hinges on the unanswered empiric issue of influence, I think it prudent to act as though gifts have their intended effects.

The third ethical consideration is the physician's character. Physicians' characters are defined by how we respond to what Al Jonsen has described as the "profound moral paradox" in which we all live, the constant balancing of altruistic concern for others–responding to an emergency call, sacrificing sleep or leisure to serve a patient's needs–and our innate self-interest and ambition (9). We all recognize this incessant tension between altruism and self-interest. The balance is precarious, however. Situations that promote our self-indulgence without considering our patients' welfare may tip the balance between self-interest and altruism, thereby altering our characters. Gifts from drug companies feed our human tendencies toward self-interest; they rarely foster our concern for our patients.

The prevalence of gifts, their effects, and their ethical implications suggest that guidelines are needed. Justice, physicians' special relationship with patients, and a proper balance between altruism and self-interest are regulative ideals, but we do not always achieve our ideals. Principles and guidelines may not only clarify uncertain situations and reduce our discomfort over the present free-for-all, but hopefully, they will also promote our quest to achieve our ideals. I suggest five such guidelines.

First, the issue should be acknowledged. In the past year, many professional organizations have made statements on this issue for the first time–the American College of Physicians (ACP), the American College of Cardiology, and the American Medical Association (AMA), among others. But recognition of the ethical dangers inherent in our accepting gifts is sometimes limited. For example, the ACP states that gifts in themselves are not the issue (10). In considering the influence of gifts, the ACP ignores their injustice. In the future, we should recognize that gifts *are* the issue.

Second, the obligations of gifts should be minimized. This principle is at the heart of the positions of both the ACP and the AMA. The ACP position is that "gifts, hospitality, or subsidies offered to physicians by the pharmaceutical industry ought not to be accepted if acceptance might influence or appear to others to influence the objectivity of clinical judgment" (10). The AMA position is that "gifts accepted by physicians individually should primarily entail a benefit to patients and should not be of substantial value" (11).

According to these professional organizations, some fruit are allowed. Inexpensive educational gifts such as books and modest meals are okay. The AMA also endorses gifts related to work, and the ACP approves funding for trips to educational sites chosen for convenience and not pleasure. Other fruit are forbidden, such as cash or the winter conference in Montego Bay. However, I must question these lists. Are they really compatible with the principles espoused by the ACP and the AMA? When is the last time any of us saw an inexpensive medical text, and do we really believe that even a modest meal for physicians benefits our patients? Is it not likely that a well-conducted CME course with a topic or speakers selected by a company might "influence the objectivity of our clinical judgment"?

Moreover, the litany of acceptable fruit ignores the importance of the gift relationship itself. The key here is not the monetary value of the gift, but whether it is instrumental in fostering a personal gift relationship. I suggest that if drug company gifts are accepted at all, they should be direct contributions to physicians' education or to patient care, and they should be made in ways that explicitly avoid the relationship or obligation of the physician to the drug company or its representative. These contributions could be channeled through nonprofit institutions such as foundations, professional societies, or academic departments. The institution that functions as middleman has ethical responsibilities as well, of course, but the subtle threat to the individual physician's character and duty to his or her patient is minimized by avoiding a personal relationship and its attendant obligations.

Clearly, the simplest solution is to just say "no." It is, perhaps, a reflection of the magnitude of the problem that the usual response to this suggestion from our colleagues is a look stating, "You must be crazy." One common response is, "I could stop at any time, but the gifts are all around, they're trivial, and you don't really believe they have any influence, do you?" (This response is reminiscent of a garrulous and unreformed alcoholic.) A second response is, "I could stop at any time, but it would cost me (my fellowship funding, uncommitted research dollars, or ability to host CME events), and you don't really believe they have any influence, do you?" In the immediate future, "Just say no" is no more likely to win the battle of gifts than it is to win other wars. Any steps in this direction will require a national effort. The first two principles are that the issue of gifts must be acknowledged and that obligations should be minimized.

The third principle is that of disclosure. While potential conflicts of interest are inevitable for each of us, they are more acceptable-and at least open to discussion-if our patients and colleagues are aware of them. As I have suggested, however, disclosure is not always practical, and even disclosure does not rectify an improper action. Our British colleagues cleverly suggest that we use this criterion: ". . . would you be willing to have these arrangements generally known(12)?" I would argue that although an answer of "no" certainly suggests a problem, an answer of "yes" does not mean that an action is above ethical question. We should recognize that disclosure may be necessary but not sufficient.

The fourth principle applies to the special case of continuing medical education, which must be free from commercial influence. The ACP, AMA, and other organizations endorse this principle but recognize that much education is underwritten by drug companies. It is widely acknowledged that influence is likely by selective support of certain topics and specific speakers. It seems strange that physicians, with their average income in six figures and their dedication to staying up-to-date, need their educational efforts underwritten at all. In the future, the most straightforward solution would be to separate the selection of topic, speakers, and audience from the support of education. Drug companies could make contributions for the support of education to an independent national organization, such as the Commonwealth Foundation.

Finally, we must acknowledge our responsibilities to our students and junior colleagues. Currently, the topic is taboo. We must begin a dialogue in our teaching and act according to our principles. We should discuss the ethical dangers inherent in relationships with drug companies and their representatives and emphasize the importance of critical consideration of primary data and expert recommendations in the choice of drugs. At the very least, these interactions should be discussed in the same formal, problem-oriented manner in which we teach about heart failure, cirrhosis, and alcoholism. Handling the topic of drug marketing with the time-honored "see one, do one, teach one" approach is not appropriate.

I conclude that as individuals, physicians should avoid accepting gifts from drug companies. Patients' money is spent unfairly. Gifts may threaten the physician-patient relationship by altering our prescribing practices. Gifts may also shift the balance between altruism and self-interest. The medical profession should structure its relationship with the drug industry according to its principles and patients' best interests.

REFERENCES

1. Chren MM, Landefeld CS, Murray TH. Doctors, drug companies, and gifts. JAMA 1989;262:3448-51.

2. Shaughnessy AF. Drug promotion in a family medicine training center. JAMA 1988;260:926.

3. Avorn J, Chen M, Hartley R. Scientific versus commercial sources of influence on the prescribing behavior of physicians. Am J Med 1982;73:4-8.

4. Lurie N, Rich EC, Simpson DE, et al. Pharmaceutical representatives in

academic medical centers: interaction with faculty and housestaff. J Gen Intern Med 1990;5:240-3.

5. Goldfinger SE. A matter of influence. N Engl J Med 1987;316:1408-9.

6. Mauss M, Cunnison I, trans. The gift: forms and functions of exchange in archaic societies. New York: W. W. Norton & Co. Inc., 1967.

7. Emerson RW. Gifts. In: Essays of Ralph Waldo Emerson. Norwalk, CT: Easton Press, 1979:211-4.

8. Fakes RW. Doctors and the drug industry. Br Med J 1986;293:1170-1.

9. Jonsen AR. Watching the doctor. N Engl J Med 1983;308:1531-5.

10. Goldfinger SE, American . . . Committee. Physicians and the pharmaceutical industry. Ann Intern Med 1990;112:624-6.

11. Council on Ethical and Judicial Affairs of the American Medical Association. Gifts to physicians from industry. JAMA 1991;265:501.

12. The relationship between physicians and the pharmaceutical industry: a report of the Royal College of Physicians. J R Coll Physicians Lond 1986; 20: 235-42.

The Need for Guidelines in Pharmaceutical Promotion: A Pharmacy Perspective

John A. Gans

When I received the invitation to be a part of the Ohio Pharmaceutical Seminar, I was not overly excited about the subject matter. It was not that the subject of pharmaceutical promotion is not important–of course it is. Pharmaceutical promotion has been the focus of much attention over the years, and it is certainly a topic that affects pharmacists and their patients. But to tell you the truth, I did not think that the subject of pharmaceutical promotion was an especially timely one.

But it was not long after the invitation arrived that it became apparent that the subject was going to become a very timely topic indeed. Prior to that time, there had been some murmuring on Capitol Hill about excesses in pharmaceutical promotion, but it was not until last December that Senator Edward Kennedy announced that he was launching a series of hearings on abuses by the pharmaceutical industry. Also in December, the new Food and Drug Administration (FDA) Commissioner, David Kessler, in his very first speech, cited prescription drug marketing as one of the items on his priority list of hot issues facing the FDA. It became very clear that whether the industry liked it or not, pharmaceutical promotion *would* become a very timely issue and that the organizers of this seminar were right on target. Not only is the subject of pharmaceutical promotion a timely topic, but it is also a complex one. This seminar is evidence of that fact. We have heard from a long list of experts, each addressing a different perspective on this controversial issue.

The American Pharmaceutical Association (APhA) is gratified that as the national professional society of pharmacists we were asked to provide pharmacy's perspective on the promotion issue at this seminar. Even so,

John A. Gans, Pharm.D., is Executive Vice President of the American Pharmaceutical Association, 2215 Constitution Avenue, NW, Washington, DC 20037.

I must admit that the assignment made me nervous. The reason is that I am not sure that there *should* be a pharmacy perspective on this issue. It seems to me that there should be just one perspective that guides all policy and action related to pharmaceutical promotion, and that is the *patient's* perspective. It is the patient who must be the driving force here. The patient's perspective must be the industry's perspective, it must be the prescriber's perspective, and yes, it must be pharmacy's perspective.

APhA recently has developed a mission statement for the profession of pharmacy, and the focus of that mission statement is not the pharmacist: it is the patient. APhA's mission statement for the profession of pharmacy is: ''The mission of pharmacy is to serve society as the profession responsible for the appropriate use of medications, devices and services to achieve optimal therapeutic outcomes.'' The focus of that statement is quite clear. The goal of all of us, whether it be the manufacturers, the regulators, the prescribers, or the dispensers, must be to assure that the patient who receives medication receives the maximum therapeutic outcome from its use. It is the patient–not the manufacturer, not the prescriber, not the pharmacist–who must be the ultimate beneficiary.

This is not a new concept. Over the past two decades or so, it has become increasingly clear to all health professionals and to the public at large that patients must play a prominent role in their own health care. Patients no longer blindly trust their physicians to provide the right care. They want to have a say in deciding what that care should be. Patients are no longer content to accept a mysterious, anonymous medication prescribed with scant explanation by their physicians and dispensed with little or no information by their pharmacists. They want to know what is wrong with them, what treatment options are available, what medication is being prescribed for them and why, whether there are any risks involved, and complete information about how to use that medication properly.

Further, consumers are taking a greater interest in self-care, and they want the right kind of information–information that will help them carry out their self-care role safely and effectively. As the self-care movement grows and the sophistication of the consumer increases, there is going to be even more responsibility placed on all of us to assure that consumers get the kind of information that they want and need.

This is not a new issue for the American Pharmaceutical Association. Most of the policies that our association has adopted in recent years and most of the activities in which we have been involved have a common root. They stem from the profession's recognition that pharmacy must be an information-based profession dedicated to serving patients and assuring that they use their medication safely and effectively. For example, in 1977, APhA adopted a policy on communicating drug information to patients that included the following:

1. Patients have the right to be informed participants in decisions related to their health care.
2. Pharmacists have a professional obligation to contribute to the education of patients to achieve optimal drug therapy.

Few can argue about the patient's need for good information or about the responsibility of all of us to provide it. But the issue gets murkier when we begin to examine the subject of this seminar, pharmaceutical promotion. The basic question, of course, is whether the message used in promotion is actually information, or is it something else? And if promotion is information, is it the kind of information that patients need to make informed decisions about their own health care? But most important, if consumers are not getting the kind of information they need, how can we work better together to see that they do?

But much of the controversy surrounding this issue, and the thing which has especially piqued the interest of the federal government, has little to do with the quality of information. Instead, many of the promotional practices now under fire are alleged to have nothing to do with information at all. They are under attack because many of them are viewed simply as attempts to promote drug use by giving gifts and incentives. Senator Kennedy and Commissioner Kessler simply do not believe that many of these promotional practices by manufacturers can be considered as providing unbiased information upon which informed and rational therapeutic decisions can be made.

Much of the criticism about pharmaceutical promotion has been directed thus far toward the relationship that exists between the pharmaceutical industry and the medical profession, and in fact, it has been that relationship that has usually felt the heat over the years. So far, the pharmacy profession has been relatively untouched by any accusations of impropriety. That does not necessarily mean that pharmacists are more ethical than physicians. It simply means that for many years, the industry has viewed the prescriber–not the pharmacist–as the primary decision maker in the drug use process. It always was the prescriber who made the choice about what drug product to use. There was very little role in the decision-making process for the pharmacist and certainly even less for the patient. It was simply good business to direct most promotional activities toward physicians rather than pharmacists.

That situation is changing now. With the advent of drug product selection laws, the increasing influence of pharmacy and therapeutics committees in the institutional setting, the increased number of pharmacy buying groups, and the promise of growth in the importance of pharmacy-centered drug utilization review programs in all health care settings, the pharmacist is becoming more than just a bystander in the decision-making process. Consequently, as the pharmacist becomes an even more prominent player, promotional activities directed at pharmacists undoubtedly will increase.

For the moment, however, current criticism has been directed primarily at the industry and the medical profession. To their credit, both have responded. The American Medical Association, the American College of Cardiology, the American College of Physicians, and the Pharmaceutical Manufacturers Association have recently adopted guidelines for their members designed to help them to avoid situations in which promotional activities might be considered unethical, or at least questionable. Some of these corrective actions have undoubtedly come about directly because of the current government scrutiny of the promotional activities of the pharmaceutical industry. But it should not go unnoticed that many pharmaceutical manufacturers dealt with these issues long before the current heat began to be felt. Many companies have, for some time, had guidelines to govern their advertising and promotional activities.

One thing that we must keep in perspective in these troubled times is that advertisement and promotion are not inherently bad for consumers/patients. Advertising and promotion are characteristic of our free enterprise system. Pharmacies and hospitals engage in it. Even lawyers and health professionals now do so. If it were not for advertising, the print and electronic media could not survive. But these benefits accrue only if advertising and promotion are used as a means of disseminating unbiased, factual, and nonmisleading information that will enable patients/consumers to make informed decisions. It was this basic premise that led to the American Pharmaceutical Association's present policy on advertising prescription drugs to the public. In 1988, when there was a considerable movement toward advertising prescription drugs to the public, one of the APhA policy committees was asked to study the issue and to recommend an association policy on the matter.

That policy did not come easily. The committee that finally recommended it did so only after considerable soul searching. There were those on the committee who felt strongly that there was absolutely no role for advertising and promotion in health care. They believed that therapeutic decisions should be made by health care professionals based on scientific information, not on promotional persuasion.

There were others who believed that advertising the availability of a new treatment for a previously untreatable condition would be a service to patients. Patients who had conditions that they believed to be untreatable could be provided information that would encourage them to seek treatment.

Finally, there were those on the committee who felt that although patients should be informed about their therapy, it should be the physician and the pharmacist who provide the information to them. Patients should not be placed in the position of making decisions on their own health care solely on the basis of promotion-slanted information. But even more important, such patients should not consult with their physicians with their minds already made up about what their condition is and what their treatment should be. Health care professionals should not be put in the position of being coerced by patients whose opinions have been shaped by promotional messages rather than scientifically based information.

The policy that resulted from the committee's debate was a compromise, and even that compromise measure was not adopted unanimously. Many delegates remained opposed to the approval of any kind of advertising of prescription drug products. Nevertheless, in the democratic body that is the House of Delegates, the compromise measure finally passed. The compromise was that although the policy would permit a drug manufacturer to advertise the availability of a new breakthrough drug, it would prohibit the use of the drug's name in the advertising, thereby–hopefully–discouraging the use of traditional advertising techniques. The policy adopted by the APhA House of Delegates is as follows:

> The American Pharmaceutical Association supports federal and state legislative and regulatory activities that would permit pharmaceutical company consumer advertising which informs patients of medical or health conditions which are treatable by prescription drug products manufactured or distributed by that company, as long as no specific reference to generic or brand names is made.

For a period of time after the passage of that policy, it appeared that it might be right on target. We did begin to see more advertising in the print and electronic media, but in accordance with the APhA policy, these ads were not advertising specific prescription drug products. They were primarily aimed at telling consumers that a new and previously unavailable treatment was now available and that they should consult their physicians for more information. But I need not tell you that the nature of prescription drug advertising has been gradually changing since that time. Specific drug names are now commonly used, and many ads are clearly aimed at touting one drug over a competing one rather than announcing the availability of breakthrough therapy.

APhA has not yet reexamined its policy on prescription drug advertising, and there are no immediate plans to do so. I would not even attempt to predict what our House of Delegates might do if we were to revisit the issue. However, I would venture this guess: if those debating the issue in 1988 could have had the benefit of the experience that we have had with prescription drug advertising since that time, the proposed policy statement might have been in a lot of trouble. It is my guess that many of the delegates who supported the APhA policy probably feel that much of the advertising we are now seeing has stepped over the boundary that the policy established.

Much of the hullabaloo about pharmaceutical promotion is not centered on advertising, however; it is focused on other kinds of promotional activities like outright gifts, payment for attending continuing education programs, and free trips to lavish continuing education seminars in exotic settings. APhA does not have an official policy on these activities. In the past, as I indicated earlier, pharmacists were not a prime target for such activities. As a result, there was never a real need to deal with the subject on an official policy level. Even so, for many years APhA has had in place informal internal policies to govern our relationship with pharmaceutical manufacturers.

First, let me make it clear that there is nothing inherently improper or unethical about pharmaceutical manufacturers supporting the activities of nonprofit professional societies that serve the professions with which manufacturers, by their nature, are intertwined. Manufacturers realize that manufacturing and distributing a quality pharmaceutical product is not sufficient to make that product therapeutically effective and of maximum benefit to the patient. To accomplish that, the product must be prescribed by a knowledgeable prescriber, and it must be dispensed by a competent pharmacist educated to help the patient realize maximum therapeutic outcomes from its use.

It is, therefore, clear that the pharmaceutical manufacturer has a large stake in seeing that the physicians and pharmacists are maximally educated and trained and that they maintain the highest practice standards. But more importantly, it is not the manufacturer or the physician or the pharmacist who is the ultimate beneficiary: it is the patient. So support of association efforts that enhance the competence of practitioners is a legitimate activity of pharmaceutical manufacturers. From the viewpoint of professional associations, it is not only legitimate, but essential to our operations. If APhA were required to limit its educational services for members to those that it could provide through member dues income, its continuing education program would be severely crippled. And, in the long run, if APhA's educational capability were lessened, the competence of the members we serve would ultimately be adversely affected.

That is not to say that there should not be guidelines set on how such support is offered and accepted. APhA and the manufacturers with whom it deals have long recognized that. As a result, we have had a long-standing policy that no manufacturer who provides financial support for an educational program shall have any control over the content of that program.

APhA's policy also attempts to prevent even the appearance of impropriety. For example, we discourage the sponsorship of programs on subjects in which manufacturers have a large financial stake, even if they exercise no control over program content. It is easy to see that many observers might consider a program on hypertension biased if it were sponsored by the manufacturer of a major hypertensive agent with a number of competitors, even though safeguards were in place to avoid bias. We help manufacturers avoid those situations by steering them to sponsorship of educational programs that carry with them no risk of such misconceptions.

I am not sure whether the charges that are currently being made about pharmaceutical promotion have merit or are just a tempest in a teapot. But the beauty of my assignment this morning is that I do not have to make that assessment. My assignment is to give pharmacy's perspective, and from pharmacy's perspective, we just do not have a major problem–at least not yet. Our goal in pharmacy, then, must be to work with pharmaceutical manufacturers to ensure that any future promotional activities involving pharmacists do not fall into question. A major step in that direction is one I mentioned earlier. We must assure that there is a clear distinction between what is promotion and what is information, and we must be sure that one is never confused with the other.

The clear objective of promotion is to sell products. But in the case of pharmaceuticals, the time-honored methods for selling more conventional merchandise simply do not apply. However, there is a clear role for information in helping to assure the maximum and effective use of pharmaceutical products. And guess what? That achieves the same objective!

Physicians are perfectly capable of recognizing a unique and effective product by reviewing scientific data about it. They should not be coerced or bribed to use it. Pharmacists have the education and training to manage effectively the use of that product by the patient if they are given straightforward and reliable information to use in doing so.

One of our mutual goals, then, should be to establish clear channels of unbiased information exchange, unfettered by promotional bias. Manufacturers should continue to support efforts to provide unbiased continuing education programming to pharmacy practitioners, and they should provide science-based information to practitioners through professional journal advertising. Manufacturers should also consider supporting organizations whose sole purpose is to enhance communication about prescription drugs among patients, physicians, pharmacists, and other health care professionals. One such organization is the National Council on Patient Information and Education. APhA, as well as other pharmacy organizations, is a charter member of this broad-based organization whose sole purpose is to foster better communications about prescription drugs.

Assuring that consumers have easy access to quality information on drug products so they can make informed decisions must be a goal for all of us. And I can think of no better way of doing that than by providing the information through qualified health professionals. APhA thinks one of the primary roles of the pharmacist should be to serve as a direct conduit to the public for drug information.

It is this philosophy–the public's need for information and the pharmacist's ability to provide it–that has led APhA to seek a new class of drugs. This new class would be a transition class into which certain drugs would pass between prescription-only status and totally unrestricted over-the-counter distribution. During that time, when the public's ability to handle these drugs properly would still be unproven, the drugs would be available only through consultation with a pharmacist. This would assure that patients choosing to self-medicate with these drugs would have full access to the information that would enable them to use the drugs safely and effectively.

There has been considerable opposition to that concept in the past, and at one time, that was understandable. Nonprescription drugs were generally very safe and uncomplicated, much more so than their prescription-only brethren. But that situation is now changing. Nonprescription drugs are no longer innocuous, especially since more and more companies are contemplating moving drug products from prescription-only to nonprescription status.

One only needs to examine the list of drugs that are being considered for nonprescription drug status to get a feel for the potential problems: Zantac®, Tagamet®, Naprosyn®, Seldane®, Clinoril®, Carafate®, Pepcid®, Flexeril®, Dolobid®, Indocin®, Rogaine®. It is difficult to conceive how the general public will be able to use drugs such as these safely and effectively without professional guidance when, up to now, they could do so only if they were under the care of a physician.

It may very well turn out that some of these switch candidates will enter into wide, unsupervised public use without patients encountering any problems, but unfortunately, we will not know that until it actually happens. We cannot predict it in advance. But the chances are just as good that some will cause severe problems when used widely without professional consultation, and unfortunately, we cannot predict that either. With a transition class of drugs, we could make that assessment much earlier and much more accurately. Pharmacists would not only provide information about proper use of the medication-how to avoid interactions with other medications and other factors-but they would also be in a position to monitor and report to the manufacturer and to the FDA any problems they observed their patients having with the drug.

This transition class of drugs would have another advantage for both the manufacturers and the public. Its existence could help to remove doubts in the minds of the FDA reviewers about whether a legend drug should be switched to a nonprescription status. If the FDA could be assured that, for a defined period of time, the use of newly switched drugs would be monitored by pharmacists and any problems would be promptly reported, the agency might be more inclined to approve the switch. This would result in *more* drugs being available on a nonprescription basis, not *fewer*, as some critics of the transition class claim. More prescription drugs could be switched to OTC status. Manufacturers and the FDA would have additional assurances that any problems related to the switch could be quickly identified and corrected. Patients would be assured of an unbiased and reliable source of information about the drugs they take. That sounds like an "everybody wins" scenario to me!

When we look at the subject of pharmaceutical promotion-no matter what vantage point from which we view it-there can really only be one perspective: the patient's perspective. Whether we are drug manufacturers, physicians, pharmacists, regulators, or others connected with health care, that is the only legitimate perspective we can take. We are *all* here to serve the patient, and that is the bottom line.

Pharmaceutical Advertising:
A Federal Trade Commission Perspective

C. Lee Peeler

I am delighted to have the opportunity to discuss the Federal Trade Commission's (FTC) present advertising enforcement program and how that program affects over-the-counter (OTC) drug advertising in particular. By way of introduction, I want to leave no doubt about the importance that the Bureau of Consumer Protection attaches to OTC drug advertising generally. In 1990 alone, consumers spent almost $10.6 billion on nonprescription drugs, and industry sources predicted a "major wave of new over-the-counter medications" in the next 5 years (1,2).

The advertising of these products is clearly of major importance. In 1990, more than $1 billion was spent on advertising OTC products (3). And by providing information that allows consumers to select medication and to treat the symptoms of minor illnesses safely and efficiently, OTC advertising can play a major positive role in keeping health care costs from rising at a time when they are already frustratingly high.

THE COMMISSION'S APPROACH
TO OTC DRUG ADVERTISING CLAIMS

With these potential benefits, however, come important responsibilities. Very few consumers, regardless of their education, have the background to make an independent judgment about claims of efficacy for

C. Lee Peeler, J.D., is Associate Director for Advertising Practices, Federal Trade Commission, Bureau of Consumer Protection, 601 Pennsylvania Avenue, NW, Suite 4002, Washington, DC 20580.

These remarks do not necessarily reflect the views of the Federal Trade Commission or any individual commissioner.

OTC products or even about the contents of the OTC products. Whether it is the ability of an ingredient to affect a particular symptom, or even whether the product really does have more of the active ingredient doctors like best, consumers must take OTC drug claims largely on faith alone.

The FTC understands that misleading, deceptive, or unsubstantiated OTC drug claims can diminish the public's confidence in the benefits of OTC products, pose a risk to consumers' health, and, in some cases, pose a risk of immediate injury to consumers. These considerations form the foundation for the FTC's enforcement efforts to assure that claims are substantiated and that consumers are not deceived in their efforts to handle their own health needs.

The cornerstone of these efforts is the commission's advertising substantiation doctrine. That doctrine requires that all advertisers have a reasonable basis for objective claims before such claims are made in advertising (4). This doctrine was first announced in the *Pfizer* case in 1972 and has served as the basis for most of the commission's advertising cases during the 1970s and 1980s. It enjoys the strong support of the advertising community and consumers and will continue to be the focus of FTC advertising enforcement during the 1990s.

SIGNIFICANT PENDING FTC ADVERTISING CASES

FTC advertising policy is largely developed on a case-by-case basis. And there are important cases pending at the commission that address each of the three basic questions faced by any advertiser:

1. What does an ad say or communicate to consumers?
2. How much substantiation is enough to support the claims made in an ad?
3. How much information has to be disclosed in an advertisement to prevent it from being deceptive by omission?

Two such pending cases involve food advertising, and one involves an over-the-counter weight-loss product. The ultimate advertising principles represented by each of these cases will be applicable to advertisers generally, so let me briefly discuss each of them.

Kraft

The first is the *Kraft* case (5). This case involves an extensive advertising campaign that we have alleged implied to consumers that a prepackaged slice of Kraft Cheese Singles® contains as much calcium as five ounces of milk. In fact, it does not. Although each slice is made from 5 ounces of milk, approximately 30-40% of the calcium in that milk is lost in processing. That fact is not in dispute. The real question addressed in the case is whether the claims alleged by the commission were ever made in the advertising.

The commission's opinion in this case, issued after two years of litigation, is important for a number of reasons. First, the *Kraft* case is one of the few recent, fully litigated advertising cases that I am aware of between a major national advertiser and any government law enforcement agency. Thus, it has served as an important test of the application of the commission's advertising policies.

Second, in the *Kraft* opinion, the commission discusses in detail its approach to ad interpretation. In a 32-page opinion upholding the staff's allegations for all but 1 of the ads challenged, the commission reviewed the ads themselves, expert testimony as to their meaning, and "copy test" data from both the commission staff and Kraft concerning consumer interpretation of the ad. A substantial portion of the trial addressed questions concerning the comparative merits of copy testing that the FTC staff had done of consumers' interpretations of the advertising and the testing Kraft had done. In fact, the record of this case probably contains more information on copy-testing methodology than most people will ever need or want to know. In the end, the commission found that the meaning of the ad was clear from a reading of the ads themselves; thus, it was not necessary to resort to extrinsic evidence. However, because extrinsic evidence was in the record, the commission also carefully reviewed that evidence and concluded that the weight of that evidence was consistent with its own reading of the advertising.

Third, although the commission did not conclude that extrinsic evidence was necessary to interpret the ads in the *Kraft* case, the decision provides useful guidance on the question of where the commission will require such evidence and where it will not. Where extrinsic evidence is necessary, the *Kraft* opinion also offers important insight as to what forms of questioning and what types of copy testing techniques the commission will find persuasive.

Also of importance to advertisers is the portion of the commission's opinion that discusses Kraft's reaction to challenges of its advertising before the commission filed its complaint. Although Kraft argued that it should have been able to rely on its predissemination testing of its advertising, which did not show that the claims were made, the commission found that Kraft, faced with a succession of warnings about potentially deceptive claims that could be implied from its ads, should have done more to determine whether its ads were conveying misleading messages. Thus, the case illustrates that under the FTC Act, the risk of miscommunication is with the advertiser and that in assessing the need for corrective action, the agency will look at the adequacy of the advertiser's response to allegations that the advertising is deceptive.

Schering

A second important case pending at the commission challenges claims made for an over-the-counter weight-loss product, Fibre Trim® (6). At one time, this product was reported as the fastest growing OTC appetite suppressant. Among the claims being challenged in this case is that the product is an effective appetite suppressant and weight-loss aid. The trial in this case was recently completed, and both sides are preparing proposed findings of fact and conclusions of law. Unlike the *Kraft* case, where the principal issue is the interpretation of the advertising, the primary question in this case is whether the claims were adequately substantiated. At issue are questions of the adequacy of the clinical testing the respondent relied on to support its claims, including questions of the methodology used, the effect of publication in peer-reviewed journals, and the extent of the respondent's obligation to consider contradictory results of other testing and to consider its own testing in the context of the overall scientific literature. The results of the litigation should provide valuable guidance to all OTC drug advertisers on many of the most fundamental issues of advertising substantiation.

Campbell Soup

The final case in this trilogy is the commission's challenge to advertising for Campbell Soup® (7). The ad promised that because certain of Campbell's soups are low in saturated fat and cholesterol, eating them could help reduce the risk of heart disease. The commission challenged those ads as deceptive because they failed to disclose that those soups are high in sodium, and diets high in sodium may increase the risk of heart disease.

Again, the question here is one of importance to all advertisers. Although the commission's 1984 opinion in the *International Harvester* case makes it clear that deception law does not require the disclosure in advertising of every fact that a consumer might find useful or interesting, the allegations in the *Campbell* case make it clear that the commission will challenge ads where the undisclosed fact is material to the specific claim being made in the ad (8). Thus, we believe it is deceptive to claim that a product is beneficial for a particular disease when, for other reasons, it could have a detrimental effect for that same disease. A settlement resolving the *Campbell* case was recently accepted by the commission and placed on the public record for comment.

Other FTC cases set forth the advertiser's obligation to disclose information when failure to do so could cause substantial consumer injury. For example, one case involved a water filter manufacturer that failed to disclose that the filters, while cleaning the water, also leaked a potentially cancer-causing chemical into the water. And although the FTC's approach to disclosure of information is, in some ways, narrower than the Food, Drug, and Cosmetic Act's requirements for advertising of prescription drugs, it is much stricter in another way. Once the commission determines that the failure to disclose information would make the ad deceptive, the commission demands *not* just that the information be physically present in the ad, but that it be communicated to consumers. If the FTC Act requires that the information be disclosed, simply burying it in a fine print notice or placing it in an ineffective video disclaimer will not suffice (5).

FTC ACTIONS INVOLVING OTC FRINGE PRODUCTS

Many of the commission's actions in the OTC drug advertising area involve what I would describe as fringe products; that is, baldness cures, impotence remedies, bee pollen, and similar products that have been the subject of the commission's actions for many years.[1] Indeed, the legislative history of the FTC Act shows that the need to control claims for these types of products was one of the express reasons for creation of the commission's consumer protection authority in 1938 (9). Ineffective diet products and gadgets have been a persistent concern in this area. In 1989, Americans spent over $32 billion on diet products and services, and the market is expected to be over $50 billion in 1995. More than 20 million Americans are on a diet at any given time (10). As those who have followed our activities in the past know, weight-loss products have always been and continue to be an area of emphasis for the commission. In fact, the commission brought its first diet case in 1927 and has been bringing them ever since (11). Recent cases in this area have ranged from challenging amino acid products that claim to make consumers lose weight while they sleep to challenging Fat Magnets® that allegedly break into thousands of particles, each acting like a tiny magnet, attracting and trapping fat particles before flushing them out of the consumer's body (12,13).

But perhaps my favorite case in the area of health claims involves ads by American Life Nutrition, a company that advertised alleged benefits of B-Pollen® in Chinese language newspapers (14). These ads, when translated, claimed that B-Pollen can be used to prevent or treat diseases and conditions including breast cancer or heart disease, diabetes, rubella, arthritis, colds, tuberculosis, rheumatism, asthma, hay fever, kidney disease, insomnia, arteriosclerosis, constipation, hemorrhoids, high blood pressure, cerebral apoplexy, and low sex drive. This was obviously either a very effective and powerful drug or an ad that someone did not expect the government to read.

When the commission believes such advertising is not merely unsubstantiated but dishonest or fraudulent as well, it increasingly is seeking temporary restraining orders and freezes on assets for eventual return to consumers. In the Dream Away® diet pill case, we returned $1.1 million to consumers. And in a recent settlement, an infomercial producer named Twin Star Productions established a $1.5 million redress fund for buyers of its diet, baldness, and impotence products (15). The Fat Magnet case that I mentioned earlier was settled for $750,000. In addition, the Postal Service and U.S. Attorneys' offices have been aggressively seeking mail and wire fraud indictments for such products as the Cal Ban 3000® weight-loss pill (16).

A more recent concern in this area, as raised by the medical community and some congressional subcommittees, has been the advertising and marketing of nationwide weight-loss clinics. By promoting weight-loss programs that claim medical supervision, these ads may suggest a greater legitimacy to consumers. We are investigating whether these medical supervisors are properly trained and what role they play in the programs. In addition, we are investigating diet programs that advocate and promote very rapid weight loss. Where claims are made, the FTC is concerned that they be substantiated and that the weight loss not be so sudden that it poses serious undisclosed health risks.

We are also concerned that the advertising does not convey a false message to consumers that rapid weight loss is synonymous with permanent weight loss. In September, the commission filed a district court complaint challenging the representations made by one multistate diet program (17). In that case, the commission is seeking permanent injunctions against deceptive claims as well as redress in the form of refunds to consumers. This case also challenges the use of two products as part of the diet program. One, a drug named Synthroid®, has been called ineffective by the Food and Drug Administration (FDA) when given in low doses. The FDA says it is unsafe in high doses. The other, an amino acid product called growth hormone releaser, we have alleged is simply ineffective.

COMPLIANCE PROGRAM

Another important, if less visible, area of FTC involvement with drug advertising is our order compliance activity. In fact, those of you who review ads should remember that one important reason for counseling your marketing department not to become involved with the commission in the first place is that FTC orders generally do not go simply to the particular claims challenged in advertising, but through "fencing in" provisions run broadly to similar claims for other, sometimes even all, of a company's products.

Our Division of Enforcement is engaged in a review of the compliance reports for four major OTC drug manufacturers. This process recently led to the filing of a district court complaint and acceptance of a consent judgment providing for $375,000 in penalties against Sterling Drug in June 1990 (18). I would hasten to add, however, that the matter was settled and that the consent judgment does not constitute an admission by stating that the law had been violated.

In the *Sterling Drug* case, the commission alleged, among other things, that Sterling lacked adequate substantiation for muscle relaxant claims made for one of the active ingredients in Midol® and Maximum Strength Midol®. In addition to the cramp relief claims for Midol and Maximum Strength Midol, staff members also challenged Sterling's claims for another active ingredient, pyrilamine maleate, in the reformulated Original Midol® and Maximum Strength Midol Multi-Symptom Formula®. This ingredient was claimed to relieve water retention, and, again, the staff alleged that the claim was unsubstantiated. Finally, the complaint challenged Spanish language print and broadcast advertising alleging that Maximum Strength Midol PMS® would provide complete relief from all symptoms of premenstrual syndrome.

The *Sterling* case is important for what it says about the relationship of the FDA's monograph process to the commission's case selection. The claims for both ingredients challenged in this case were subject to an ongoing FDA monograph review process. In 1988, the FDA tentatively concluded that there was insufficient evidence to conclude that either ingredient was safe and effective. Although the FDA has still not finalized that decision, the FTC believed that there were sufficient grounds to challenge the claims. However, prior to 1988, one of the ingredients (pyrilamine maleate) had been tentatively classified as safe and effective; therefore, for this ingredient, the FTC challenged only claims made after the 1988 reclassification.

In summary, then, the *Sterling* case is yet another example that, although the FTC gives great deference to FDA conclusions concerning the safety and efficacy of OTC products, the mere fact of a pending FDA monograph review does not offer an advertiser a safe harbor to make unsubstantiated claims in advertising.[2]

The *Sterling* case also illustrates an important distinction between FTC enforcement and private cases under the Lanham Act, where failure to comply with FDA requirements may not result in legal liability unless the private plaintiff also can prove the claim to be false.[3]

AREAS OF FUTURE FTC INVOLVEMENT WITH OTC DRUG ADVERTISING

But the key question that many have goes beyond recent or pending cases and asks how to predict what future investigations and cases the FTC will initiate. What, then, are we looking for in the area of drug advertising?

After determining that an ad is false, misleading, or unsubstantiated, the most basic criterion we look to is the amount of consumer injury caused by the advertising. We make this assessment based on a variety of common-sense factors. For example, one of our first questions is whether the product is a fraud. There has been plenty to do in this area lately, but we believe strongly that if we expect major drug manufacturers to adhere strictly to the high standards both we and the FDA believe are necessary, we must be willing to go after ads for obviously ineffective products. And as I indicated earlier, we have frequently taken action against this type of advertising in the past and will continue to do so in the future.

One interesting issue that has arisen in these cases is instances in which the FDA approves a prescription drug for a problem for which there was previously no effective remedy. Because of statutory restrictions on brand-name advertising, prescription drug advertising could actually reinforce the credibility of unsubstantiated claims for other products. Consumers could think: "There is something out there that works. Maybe this is it." This raises yet another issue that must be considered in our case selection process.

Second, the degree of potential risk to the user's health is a very important factor. Many of the cases we select involve concerns about both efficacy and safety. Thus, diet products advertised as "100% safe," exercise devices that may break and cause serious injury, and weight-loss plans promoting prescription drugs that have not been found safe and effective for weight loss have all been targeted for commission action (13,17,19).

Third, we look at whether the claims involved are the type the public can evaluate for themselves. In the case of most drug advertising, of course, the public must rely on the veracity of the advertiser's claims.

Fourth, we want to know if there are other mechanisms that can address the issues raised. Comparative claims in drug advertising have been a frequent subject of Lanham litigation, and such actions have reduced the need for FTC actions. Thus, we want to know if there is significant competitive injury, will the competitor bring a Lanham Act case or take the matter to the network clearance or National Advertising Division of the Better Business Bureau? If the matter has been addressed by a self-governing regulatory body, we will evaluate whether that group's disposition of the matter offers consumers sufficient protection.

Fifth, we will want to know if bringing this particular case will help clarify an important question concerning advertising law, such as the kind and amount of substantiation that is necessary. This criterion is a very important one and, in appropriate cases, can override several of the other criteria listed above. In *Sterling Drug*, for example, the commission did not claim great consumer injury or risk to health. There was certainly no suggestion of fraud. Yet the case is important because it shows the commission's resolve that high standards be followed. Clinical tests must be reliable and reach statistically significant results, and claims–even for individual ingredients–must be presented in an extremely careful manner.

Thus, we face a dual task in our OTC drug advertising program. One is to be the cop on the beat for the garden-variety marketers of bogus products who are not likely to be deterred by legalisms like ad substantiation requirements. At the same time, cases involving ads for food and drug products that are household names–like the ones I have mentioned–are needed to give your industry and others guidance about the advertising standards we think should be followed.

Finally, particularly in the area of drug advertising, we want to make sure that our actions are consistent with those of other government agencies such as the FDA. And, to the extent that other government agencies are actively pursuing certain practices, we want to know whether additional involvement by the FTC is in the public interest. In doing so, we work closely with the staff of the Food and Drug Administration and, increasingly, we communicate with state attorneys general to share information about pending investigations.

These are not radically new case selection criteria. In fact, they are consistent with those that were first outlined by the commission staff in 1975. But I wanted to review them for two reasons. First, I want to provide a sense of how we select cases we are likely to be bringing in the future. Second, we have found in the past that complaints from competitors and members of the medical community are a good source of leads for new investigations. Thus, I want to encourage the pharmaceutical industry to bring to our attention cases that may fit these criteria.

I believe the 1990s will prove to be an interesting period for drug advertising. It will be a time to judge how closely the industry has adhered to the principles laid out in the *Thompson Medical* and other decisions during the 1980s. It will also be a period to judge the impact of legal principles developed by decisions in the cases I discussed at the outset. And as the FDA completes additional monographs, as it has already done for baldness and impotence products and has promised to do for the vast majority of diet products, the FTC staff will be able to direct enforcement to other areas of drug and other advertising.

Finally, I can foresee significant new issues arising that the FTC will need to address. For example, the experience gained by the commission during the 1980s, when ibuprofen switched from prescription to OTC status, highlights the need for close coordination between the FDA and the FTC when drugs switch to nonprescription status (20). We have already met with FDA staff members on this issue, and the claims made in this area will be given careful scrutiny in the future.

I predict that the 1990s will be an active and exciting period for drug advertising at the FTC and elsewhere. We look forward to working with the drug industry to ensure that both drug advertising and our regulatory policies continue to serve the consumer.

NOTES

[1]Many of these products are being sold through infomercials, 30-minute ads that sometimes pose as serious programming. These have provided much work for the commission in the last year or two.

[2]See also *Thompson Medical* 104 F.T.C. 648, 828-829 (1984).

[3]See, for example, *Sandoz Pharmaceuticals v. Richardson Vicks*, 902 F.2d 222, 227-9 (3rd Cir. 1990).

REFERENCES

1. Communication from P. Taylor, Nonprescription Drug Manufacturers Association, 11 June 1991.

2. Health care: hospitals, drugs and cosmetics–basic analysis. Standard and Poor's Industry Surveys 1990;158(29):Sec. 1.

3. Leading National Advertisers, Inc. Ad $ Summary 1990;(Jan-Dec).

4. FTC Policy Statement Regarding Advertising Substantiation, 104 F.T.C. 648, 839 (1984), *aff'd*, 791 F.2d 189 (D.C. Cir. 1986), *cert. denied*, 479 U.S. 1086 (1987).

5. *Kraft, Inc.*, D. 9208 (complaint issued January 25, 1989), final commission opinion issued January 31, 1991, appeal now pending in the United States Court of Appeals for the Seventh Circuit.

6. *Schering Corp.*, D. 9232 (complaint issued September 22, 1989).

7. *Campbell Soup Co.*, D. 9223 (April 18, 1991, provisionally accepted consent agreement).

8. *International Harvester*, 104 F.T.C. 949, 1059-60 (1984).

9. House Committee on Interstate and Foreign Commerce. Report to Accompany S. 1077, Extension of Federal Trade Commission's Authority Over Unfair Acts and Practices and False Advertising of Food, Drugs, Devices, and Cosmetics (1937).

10. Federal Trade Commission statement delivered by Chairman Janet D. Steiger before the Subcommittee on Regulation, Business Opportunities, and Energy of the U.S. House of Representatives Committee on Small Business (March 26, 1990).

11. *McGowan Labs, Inc.*, 11 F.T.C. 125 (1927).

12. *FTC v. Kingsbridge Media & Marketing, Inc.*, No. CIV-88-0003 PHX-EHC, slip op. (D. Ariz. June 8, 1988) (Dream Away).

13. *FTC v. Allied International Corp.*, No. 90-0120 CBM (KX) (C.D. Cal. filed January 9, 1990).

14. *American Life Nutrition*, C-3310 (October 18, 1990) (consent).

15. *Twin Star Productions, Inc.*, C-3307 (October 2, 1990) (consent). A consent agreement is for settlement purposes only and does not constitute an admission of a law violation. When the commission issues a consent order on a final basis, it carries the force of law with respect to future actions. Each violation of such an order may now result in a civil penalty of up to $10,000.

16. Wall Street Journal 1990 Jul 9.

17. *Pacific Medical Clinics Management, Inc.*, No. 90-1277 GT (CM) (S.D. Cal. September 27, 1990) (preliminary injunction).

18. *United States v. Sterling Drug, Inc.*, No. CA90-1352 (D.D.C. June 21, 1990) (consent decree). The consent decree against Sterling was for settlement purposes only and did not constitute an admission by Sterling of a law violation. Consent decrees, however, have the force of law.

19. *Consumer Direct, Inc.*, D. 9236 (October 29, 1990) (consent).

20. *Walgreen Co.*, C-3214 (June 10, 1987